Prenatal Screening, Policies, and Values: The Example of Neural Tube Defects

Elena O. Nightingale, M.D., Ph.D.
Susan B. Meister, Ph.D., R.N.,
Editors

A Report of the Working Groups of Early Life and Adolescent Health Policy and of Health Promotion and Disease Prevention

Division of Health Policy Research and Education
Harvard University

Harvard University

Division of Health Policy Research and Education

Harvard Medical School
John F. Kennedy School of Government
Harvard School of Public Health

Copyright 1987 by the President and Fellows of Harvard College.

ISBN 0-674-87125-1

RG628
.P73
1987

Copy 1

Acknowledgment

The authors are deeply grateful to Dr. Pamela Talalay for her invaluable contribution to the writing and editing of this report.

This work was supported by grant #7196 to Harvard University from the Robert Wood Johnson Foundation. The opinions in this report are those of the authors and not necessarily those of the Robert Wood Johnson Foundation or of Harvard University.

Design, Typesetting and Printing: Office of the University Publisher, Harvard University

Contents

Part I
The Study

Elena O. Nightingale, M.D., Ph.D. and
Susan B. Meister, Ph.D., R.N.

Preface

Rapid development of sophisticated new techniques has vastly increased our ability to diagnose congenital disorders during the prenatal period. These technical capabilities, however, have not been matched by improvements in treatment; further, the new technologies often require complex equipment and experienced personnel. Moreover, the technological advances in this field have produced serious dilemmas for the medical profession and for society.

Analytic methods such as technology assessment, decision analysis, and cost-effectiveness analysis are often used to clarify both policy options and the rationale for choosing among these options in deciding on health policies for the public. Such analytic findings are frequently limited by methodology and availability of data. Of equal concern, the methods are often applied indiscriminately to medical problems, whether appropriate or not. Even the best possible analysis may not incorporate all of the pertinent factors or assemble the factors in an appropriate fashion.

This report focuses on prenatal diagnosis of genetic disorders and birth defects, specifically diagnosis of neural tube defects. These common congenital disorders stem from genetic and environmental factors, and have grave impacts on patient, family, and health professionals. The study described here was designed to assess the role of three analytic methods in reaching health care decisions consonant with our basic ethical and societal values. Each analytic method was applied to the prenatal diagnosis of neural tube defects.

Part I of this report discusses the findings and conclusions of each analysis, described in the second part, in the context of the major ethical dilemmas faced by patients and professionals in the application of prenatal diagnostic techniques. Part II consists of three reports—technology assessment, decision analysis, and cost-effectiveness analysis.

A. Background

Each human cell contains 46 chromosomes with a total of 50,000 to 100,000 genes distributed among them. This rich genetic heritage accounts for the high

1

variability in the members of the human race, but also allows for immense possibilities for error when gene replication occurs. Such errors can give rise to genetic diseases. It is not surprising, in view of the large number of genes, that single gene disorders in man, though individually rare, when added together, pose a major public health problem. McKusick (1983) describes more than 4,000 diseases caused by mutations in a single gene (for example, sickle cell disease, a disorder of hemoglobin). In addition to single gene disorders, abnormalities in the number, size, or configuration of whole chromosomes, or segments of chromosomes, such as in Down Syndrome, and birth defects that stem from a genetic susceptibility, such as defects in the closure of the neural tube, add to the burden of genetic illness.

1. Advances in Prenatal Diagnosis for Congenital Disorders[1]

As recently as 20 years ago, clinical genetics was relatively undeveloped. If a family already had an affected child or a clear family history of a particular disease was recognized, i.e., the diagnosis was clear and the pattern of inheritance was known, risk figures for recurrence of the condition could be estimated. The options were: not to have children, try to adopt, attempt donor insemination in appropriate cases, or take the risk of having an affected child. Since that time, genetic prenatal diagnosis has been used for many diseases. For example, by 1982 more than 40 hereditary biochemical disorders had been diagnosed *in utero* and tests for 35 others were on the horizon (Simpson et al., 1982). Diagnosis of chromosomal defects has improved dramatically with banding techniques that enable detection of defects in minute portions of chromosomes. Mapping and linkage techniques have permitted detection of single gene disorders such as Huntington's disease, even if the gene responsible for the disease has not been identified (Gusella et al., 1983). Recent advances in molecular biology will expand the range of disorders that is detectable. In theory, it should eventually be possible to use recombinant DNA techniques to isolate and characterize any human gene, and as the understanding of pathogenesis increases so, it is hoped, will the design of preventive and therapeutic interventions. The mapping of the entire human genome is now within reach, enabling linkage studies that would provide insight into the common chronic diseases, such as heart disease, with complex genetic components (Lewin, 1986).

The characteristic chromosome constitution (karyotype) of man was described in the late 1950s when effective techniques for chromosome visualization and staining were developed. In the mid-1970s, the technique of sampling amniotic fluid (amniocentesis) in the middle trimester became available. The ability to detect chromosome abnormalities cytologically made amniocentesis a rational procedure. For example, the amniotic fluid could be tested for biochemical abnormalities or the fibroblasts shed from the fetus could be grown in culture and the chromosomes could be characterized.

A collaborative study of middle trimester amniocentesis was carried out by nine medical centers and the procedure was found to be acceptably safe because less than 1% of women tested had any complications (NICHHD, 1976). Available tests for gross chromosome abnormalities and a few biochemical abnormalities, such as Tay-Sachs disease, were found to be acceptably accurate.

Techniques of staining that permit visualization of the fine structure of chromosomes, and methods of analysis for almost 100 biochemical disorders are now available. The use of restriction enzymes (enzymes that cleave DNA at specific sites) and other recombinant DNA techniques, such as radioactive genetic probes that can identify specific segments of DNA and natural variations (polymorphisms) in fragments of DNA produced by restriction enzymes, also enable prenatal detection of a rapidly growing number of genetic diseases. In addition, testing the DNA itself for abnormalities makes it possible to use fibroblasts shed by the fetus into the amniotic fluid to detect disease, no matter what differentiated organ or tissue is eventually involved in the disease process. Detection is possible because the genes themselves, rather than gene products, are being probed and all cells contain the same genes. This is particularly advantageous because before DNA-specific technologies were developed sickle cell disease, for example, could be diagnosed prenatally only by removing a sample of fetal blood, a procedure with a high risk of fetal death. Disorders that became diagnosable with newer techniques include Duchenne muscular dystrophy, phenylketonuria (PKU), or disorders of the clotting system—for example, hemophilia due to Factor VIII or IX deficiency.

Research in the past two or three years has also resulted in techniques for sampling the cells of the villi of the chorion, a tissue of fetal origin that forms the placenta (Modell, 1985). The chorionic villi can be reached through a cannula inserted in the cervix, in contrast to amniocentesis, an invasive procedure that involves penetration of the mother's abdominal wall and of the amniotic sac around the fetus by a needle. Most important, chorionic villi can be sampled in the first trimester of pregnancy. If parents choose to interrupt the pregnancy, the procedure is much simpler and safer in the first trimester than in the second. If the fetus is found to be unaffected, the period of anxious waiting is much shorter.

The major risk of first trimester villus sampling is spontaneous abortion after the procedure. The extent of the risk is still being determined although the procedure is already available in a variety of centers and practice settings in the United States, Italy, the People's Republic of China, and other countries. As the procedure becomes widely used, practical problems of availability of trained personnel and laboratories and ethical problems of access or use for gender selection will become apparent.

Advances in another technique, diagnostic ultrasonography, enable visualization of fetuses so that structural defects can be diagnosed with accuracy.

Although in a few instances intrauterine treatment is possible, the choices for action when a defect is detected—by ultrasonography or other means—are usually two: allow the pregnancy to proceed with preparation for the birth of an affected child, or terminate. Yet often the diagnosis is qualitative but not predictive of the quality of life, or the degree of disability. For Tay-Sachs disease (detectable by a chemical test), whose victims inevitably die before the age of 4 or 5 years after much suffering and anguish, the implications of parental choices are fairly clear. But what of the diagnosis through amniocentesis of XXX, XXY, or XYY karyotype? Further, what of the diagnosis by ultrasonography of an abnormality of a kidney that might be repaired surgically, or of a type of dwarfism that is compatible with life, or a neural tube defect of moderate size in which total effects cannot be predicted? If a prenatal test for a severe condition becomes available, who should have the test? When are mass screening programs warranted? How can we guard against discriminatory uses of new genetic testing regimens and of their future societal abuse? (Lappe, 1984).

The pace of the advances in prenatal diagnosis of congenital disorders has been more rapid than had been thought possible. Not surprisingly, some of these advances, although they open up possibilities of a myriad of early diagnoses, also are costly and pose grave dilemmas. In the prenatal period, for such conditions, the expected gap between diagnostic and therapeutic capability is unusually wide. Nevertheless, the development of methods to detect genetic disease and other congenital disorders may lead to means of prevention or treatment.

Advances in prenatal diagnosis are, and will continue to be, rapid. Although they produce complex and compelling dilemmas, these advances are not often the subject of comprehensive policy analysis. Decisions on these matters are required in timely fashion, but well-balanced analyses are needed to prevent rapid but ill-considered choices.

The rapidly increasing technical ability to diagnose a variety of disorders before birth challenges both current concepts of medical practice and basic societal values. As the technologies enabling diagnosis develop, the associated implications for health policy become increasingly complex, particularly for mass application if it is to remain sensitive to individual values.

2. Prenatal Diagnosis and Service Delivery

Technologies for prenatal diagnosis are usually developed to identify, during the prenatal period, those congenital disorders that present serious threats to the fetus. Technologic advances have been remarkably rapid in the past 15 years since the discovery of recombinant DNA techniques. In parallel with increasing capability, demand for services will increase and is likely to grow faster than the ability to provide quality services. This situation will require difficult choices.

Until the mid-1970s, use of genetic services was generally limited to those persons who were near a major academic medical center, were aware that genetic services existed, were able to pay for the service, or could be included in a research protocol (Sepe et al., 1982). In 1976, the National Genetic Diseases Act (PL 94-278) resulted in federal funding for genetic service programs in 34 states. Although the volume of prenatal diagnosis in these states was large—42,003 amniotic fluid specimens and 3,158,521 specimens for screening of inborn errors of metabolism were tested—fewer than half of the pregnant women for whom genetic services would have been medically indicated were actually treated (Sepe et al., 1982). Since the tests in question often require highly trained personnel to obtain and analyze the specimens, the associated cost and manpower are large.

Advanced maternal age is one of the most common indications for genetic services because there is an associated risk of chromosomal disorders in children of older women. Pregnancy in women over 35 is considered to be an indication for amniocentesis. In 1979, about 2.4% of all pregnant women in New York state had amniocentesis—a 49% increase over use in 1978 (Hook et al., 1981). Grouping the women by age establishes, as expected, a sharp difference in usage: 28.7% for women over 35 years of age versus 0.54% for women under 35 years of age. Current trends toward older age for the first pregnancy suggest that the need for genetic services may increase. Adams, Oakley, and Marks (1982) project a 37% increase in the percentage of births to women over 35 during this decade. If half of these women request prenatal chromosomal diagnosis, about 1.1 million women would be seeking these services over the decade. Furthermore, if screening for neural tube defects (or any other defect, for that matter) becomes more widely accepted, the demand for services will increase even more dramatically. Hobbins et al. (1982) have suggested expanding the screening protocol for neural tube defects to include two sets of ultrasonographic examination; such developments will add a further demand for services.

4

Clearly, prenatal diagnosis has great potential for benefit. For example, more than 95% of all diagnostic results indicate that the suspected condition is not present. Thus, prenatal diagnosis most often permits couples at risk for a serious disorder to continue the pregnancy without fear. On the other hand, most rare disorders first appear in families with no history of, or other reasons to be concerned about, congenital problems. These families are not likely to use prenatal diagnosis. Therefore, whereas prenatal diagnostic technologies present new vistas for enhancing health, they also present some complex problems. Utilization is uneven. Access to services may not always be equitable or fair. The disorders that threaten health are individually relatively rare and often affect unsuspecting families. Use of the technologies requires a wide range of professional services and equipment. The challenge is to determine how best to provide the appropriate services to the largest number of women in the most just manner.

The asynchrony between technical advances and planning for delivery of services is, in part, a function of the complexity and rapid development of the field. First, as research continues, greater efforts will be required to prepare and use new knowledge effectively. Otherwise, as happened with the early screening programs for sickle cell disease, new technologies will be applied with inadequate preparation and inappropriate enthusiasm and may become widespread too quickly, sometimes causing harm (National Academy of Sciences, 1975). The effects of such errors could be potentiated in times of financial hardship, because launching the programs is expensive and may keep funds from other services of proven value.

Second, applications might threaten equitable distribution of the benefits of new knowledge. Fairness in availability and use of existing prenatal diagnostic services—and of new ones as they are developed—is an important issue since there is marked racial disparity in early use of routine prenatal care, a prerequisite for prenatal diagnosis. Data from the National Center for Health Statistics for 1981, the most recent available at this writing, reveal that more black women do not obtain prenatal care until after the first trimester than is the case for white women (Figure 1). Women with delayed or no prenatal care are automatically excluded from consideration for prenatal diagnosis. Plans to apply prenatal diagnostic technologies must include consideration of these preexisting disparities in access to and use of basic prenatal services. These plans require removal of barriers that contribute to disparity, such as those stemming from cultural, social, educational, economic, access, or language factors, which themselves have several ramifications (Murray et al., 1980). For example, economic factors include more than the ability to pay, since plans for reimbursement affect the organization of services. If services are not reimbursed, they may not be offered, which ultimately makes the ability to pay a moot point. Even if early prenatal care is sought and obtained, awareness of genetic and other congenital disorders and what can be done about them may be lacking.

Third, applications of prenatal technologies should be considered in the context of changes in related technologies. For example, neonatal intensive care has also advanced rapidly in the last decade. As survival of smaller and younger fetuses becomes possible—now a fairly routine occurrence for those born weighing less than 1,000 grams—the time for termination of affected pregnancies will be reduced, as will the time available for prenatal diagnosis. Currently, termination of a pregnancy is allowed at 24 weeks, but soon survival may be possible at 24 weeks. Although the risk of major disability increases with decreasing age and size of surviving premature babies, the possibility of earlier survival requires reevaluation

5

Figure 1

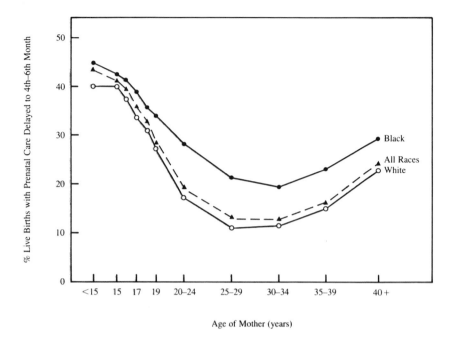

Utilization of Prenatal Care. Percent of Live Births with Prenatal Care Beginning in 4th–6th Month. Based on 100 percent of births in selected states and on a 50 percent sample of births in all other states. From: National Center for Health Statistics: Advance report of final natality statistics, 1981. Monthly Vital Statistics Report Vol. 32, No. 9. Supp DHHS Pub. No. (PHS) 84-1120. Public Heatlh Service. Hyattsville, MD. Dec. 1983.

of policies on prenatal diagnosis and selective abortion. Abortion can be accepted as an option only at a time in gestation when extrauterine survival would not be possible. In addition to technical considerations, restrictions on reimbursement for or reversal of the legality of abortion will sharply reduce options for dealing prenatally with severely handicapping conditions.

Advances in other techniques for prenatal diagnosis are also pertinent. For example, prenatal diagnosis in the first trimester by chorionic villus biopsy is becoming widely available (Cowart, 1983; Modell, 1985). First trimester diagnosis will make decisions about termination easier for many, but will make diagnosis more inaccessible to others, such as women delaying prenatal care until after the first trimester of pregnancy. As shown in Figure 1, very young women and black women are more likely to fall into this group.

Another example is provided by measurement of maternal serum alpha-fetoprotein (MSAFP), a test used for prenatal diagnosis of neural tube defects (NTDs). Higher than normal levels of MSAFP can indicate an NTD in the fetus. Recently, it has been reported that abnormally low levels of this substance are indicative of a chromosome disorder, Down Syndrome (Cuckle and Wald, 1984). This finding changes the assessment of the value of MSAFP screening and the likelihood of its becoming widely used. The American College of Obstetricians and Gynecologists has issued a professional liability alert for MSAFP screening both for Down Syndrome and for NTDs (ACOG, 1985). The prospect of liability for not screening has placed routine MSAFP screening on their docket for this decade.

All of these issues bear upon decisions to use prenatal diagnostic technologies. The breadth of knowledge that can be applied is important because the decisions to be made are extremely diverse. For example, decisions range from determining how to use prenatal diagnostic technologies for an individual fetus to deciding how best to use them for the larger population. But, as illustrated above, a number of considerations other than factual knowledge may influence the decision.

By using the time of diagnosis (i.e., prenatal or postnatal) and the options for the treatment, congenital disorders can be grouped into at least four major categories:

1. Major problems for which no treatment is available and termination of pregnancy would be medically indicated (e.g., anencephaly, some trisomies);
2. Major problems for which palliative or symptomatic treatment or management is available. Treatment may be intrauterine, e.g., hydrocephalus (very rare), or postnatal, e.g., neural tube defects;
3. Major problems for which obtaining information and treatment could be deferred until birth without changing the outcome (e.g., cleft palate and other structural defects);
4. Boundary problems with insufficient knowledge to determine action (e.g., XYY karyotype).

A categorization such as this would help to clarify thinking and would aid decision making. For example, screening for conditions in categories 3 and 4 would be ill-advised except perhaps for research purposes (National Academy of Sciences, 1975). Patients with conditions in categories 1 and 2 would be candidates for possible screening. Specific disorders may move from one class to another as the ability to diagnose improves, the disease is understood better, or treatments become available. For example, the implications of the XXX and XXY chromosome constitution are becoming clearer (S. Walzer, personal communication). Soon these conditions might move from category 4 to category 2 because early treatment of associated learning disabilities is proving effective. However, the implications of XYY are still poorly understood so for now this condition remains a boundary problem. Considering the whole array of implications would eventually provide a basis for guidelines on what actions should be taken.

3. Use of Health Policy Analysis

Analysis of health policy options can bring scientific advances to bear upon health problems so that the rationale for the chosen course of action is clear, and the choices made are as sound as possible. Policies can be developed so that new tools are effectively, efficiently, and equitably applied. The use of policy analysis to protect and promote health has special implications for children. Selection of appropriate policies is especially important to the welfare of any group that lacks power, because the policies can serve to protect the interests of the group.

In the field of prenatal diagnosis, patients, providers, and others, such as lawmakers, become involved in judgments about highly personal decisions, such as abortion. Thus, decisions become complicated and subject to public scrutiny and actions. It is not appropriate simply to apply available scientific findings to the decisions because data are seldom complete and because automatic application of scientific discoveries can cause problems if the full array of implications for the individual patient and for the population is not considered.

Decisions in accord with the values of our society might begin with analysis of the quality and appropriateness of the knowledge that can be used. However, scientific findings are most useful if they are applied together with other kinds of information. Richmond and Holtzman (1983) suggest several steps: increase knowledge of the public and providers; create processes to pilot test technologies before policies are enacted; and develop mechanisms that allow all points of view to be heard.

Construction of health policies should depend on analyses (technical and of moral values) of how to make best social use of knowledge and resources (Pellegrino, 1985). Several forms of technical analysis, although not ends in themselves, when taken together can assist in clarifying thinking and delineating options. Many components of decisions relating to wide application of prenatal diagnostic techniques can be quantified, but it is essential that numbers *per se* do not supersede common sense and good judgment in making decisions both for the individual and the population at large. An appropriate knowledge base for making the decisions that produce policies is a necessary, but not a sufficient, condition. Rather, to formulate options and make the best choices, analyses should be selected to produce information that fully addresses all the pertinent issues.

The importance of analytical methods varies depending on whether they are to be used for decisions relating to individuals, facilities, or agencies. Prospective parents and health care professionals face decisions involving the well-being of someone else—the fetus, who, in turn, affects the well-being of the family—and who, in some cases, becomes a public charge. Health care systems must weigh the value of preventing or controlling genetic and congenital disease against the cost of providing highly technical, labor-intensive services. Public and private agencies must compare the benefits of investing in services for victims of such disorders against those of investing in the facilities and personnel required for their prevention or control. Society must consider the benefit of affecting the public view of prevention of genetic disorders against the risk of adversely affecting the perception of self-worth of persons with disabling disorders that could have been diagnosed prenatally and prevented by selective abortion.

When decisions to apply prenatal technologies are made, fairness and equity are difficult to uphold because of existing differences in access both to services and to information about those services. Advances in technologies are not often uniformly available to the entire population, particularly technologies that are expensive, time-intensive, and new. A group composed of persons with diverse backgrounds and experience in fields ranging from genetics, biology, medicine, nursing, obstetrics, and pediatrics to ethics, health economics, law, and psychology was formed to study these questions[2]. The results of this multidisciplinary study are discussed below, followed by full reports of the supporting technical analyses.

B. Design of the Study: Rationale and Methods

It is clear from the introduction that recent rapid advances in technology and in society's concepts of medical care in a variety of medical fields pose major problems to development of relevant health policies. This is particularly compelling in the area of prenatal diagnosis because these policies affect whole families in very

8

personal and emotionally stressful ways.

Ideally information and services need to be presented fairly so that prospective parents can make the best choices in the prevention, management, or treatment of serious birth defects. In that way parents could avoid tragedies that result when usable information is unavailable to them. For example, parents cannot choose either selective interruption of a pregnancy when the fetus is severely affected or make the best preparation for the birth of such a child unless they have appropriate information. Our study is an attempt to determine whether current analytic methods can be used to provide better information for policy development (rather than for individual decision-making directly) and, if so, how to expedite the processes. We chose three well-studied methods; technology assessment (TA), decision analysis (DA), and cost-effectiveness analysis (CEA). These techniques were applied to a specific condition, with both genetic and environmental components, namely neural tube defects, for which prenatal screening involving several tests and procedures has recently become available. We wanted to determine, by examining and analyzing data from published reports, to what extent each of the designated methods, alone or in sequence, contribute to making informed policy decisions that are consonant with the basic values of our society.

Technology assessment, decision analysis, and cost-effectiveness analysis were chosen because they are currently being used increasingly for addressing medical questions involving new techniques, uncertainties regarding whether the techniques are beneficial to entire or only to selected populations, and, if availability of effective technologies is limited, for addressing decisions about who should receive them. In particular, we wanted to know how the use of these analytic methods could support our society's values with reference to health care. This study does not provide indepth ethical analyses; instead, we elected to examine several widely agreed upon principles of bioethics for health care in conjunction with the analytic methods (Beauchamp, 1982; Veatch, 1981).

Ethical questions about various aspects of the delivery of health care, genetic screening, and prenatal diagnosis have been discussed by the National Academy of Sciences (1975), the President's Commission for the Study of Ethical Problems in Medicine and Biomedical Behavioral Research (1983), subcommittees of professional clinical societies, the Hastings Center (Powledge and Fletcher, 1979), the Kennedy Institute on Bioethics, the Council for International Organizations of Medical Sciences (Pellegrino, 1985), and others. Although the groups use different methods and study different issues, their analyses demonstrate the pertinence of values and ethics to health care, genetic screening, and prenatal diagnosis.

We reviewed the work of the President's Commission for the Study of Ethical Problems in Medicine and Biomedical and Behavioral Research and drew upon their findings. The Commission identified three basic ethical principles that were essential requirements in providing health care (President's Commission, 1983). These are well-being, autonomy, and equity. They provide the framework for our discussion of societal values and are defined below.

The principle of well-being describes the basic goal of health care—to do no harm and to promote the health and welfare of people affected by health care, including the patient, family, larger community, and provider. The Commission indicated that the principle of well-being does not imply that one may only adopt a course that has no risk of harming anyone. Rather, choosing a course requires deciding when the risk of harm is justifiable in light of the probable benefits. They also commented that implications for people other than the patient (family, community, society) are increasingly important.

In the context of prenatal diagnosis, a decision may affect the well-being of the fetus, the parents, or society in different ways. For example, prenatal diagnosis may identify a fetus who would benefit from a prenatal treatment that, however, would pose an additional risk to the mother. Weighing these effects is necessary to making an ethical decision.

The principle of autonomy addresses individual freedom of choice and includes providing information to patients, honoring and supporting the choices of patients, and protecting their privacy. This principle also applies to professionals and, therefore, protects providers from being required to act in a manner contrary to their beliefs.

In the context of prenatal diagnosis, the preferred choices of parents and providers may differ. If the parents are competent, their freedom of choice prevails, although the law may constrain their range of choices. The degree to which the parent is a risk taker also enters into expressions of choice. One of the most difficult aspects of applying this principle to prenatal diagnosis arises from the necessity of one person (parent) making a choice for another (fetus). Parental responsibility for the health care of their children is not new, but advances in prenatal diagnosis present new extensions of that responsibility. Thus, ethical decisions in this field must recognize several interested parties, only some of whom can express their values and preferences. Sometimes these parties present competing or mutually exclusive preferences.

The President's Commission identified two aspects of the principle of equity in health care. In some instances, this principle implies that all people be treated equally. In other instances, the principle of equity would imply that all people be treated fairly rather than equally. Fairness sometimes supports preferential treatment for individuals with greater health needs. In other words, the principle of equity does not necessarily require that all resources be distributed equally.

The need to contain health care costs and to make difficult allocation decisions coupled with increased technologic capabilities mandates that analytic methods such as CEA will be used to guide policy. We wished to examine to what extent these methods aid decisions that are not only correct from a fiscal perspective but are also correct in terms of societal values.

The results of technology assessment are described in detail in Part II, Section A, the results of decision analysis applied to one of the screening procedures (second trimester ultrasonography) are delineated in Part II, Section B, and those of cost-effectiveness analysis in Part II, Section C.

Prenatal screening for neural tube defects was chosen as the study example for several reasons. It is now possible to offer a series of procedures to screen for NTD-affected fetuses. These include two tests for measuring levels of a fetal protein (alpha-fetoprotein) in the maternal serum, ultrasonography for visualizing the fetus, and amniocentesis to provide samples of amniotic fluid for further testing. None of these tests and procedures provides a definitive diagnosis *per se* and each may produce some false results.

Since MSAFP test kits have recently been approved by the U.S. Food and Drug Administration (FDA) for general use by physicians, but ultrasonography and amniocentesis require equipment and expertise which is less generally available, it appeared to us that screening for neural tube defects would provide a particularly

10

appropriate problem for analysis. For example, the diagnostic and screening techniques currently in use are under further development, the complete sequence of testing is relatively new, the available literature is scattered, and the information is incomplete. Further, even if prenatal testing for NTDs were completely accurate, the test results do not provide information on the ultimate function of the individual. A brief survey of the NTD literature indicated that ethics and values were rarely discussed, and if mentioned, were considered in passing. In short, the situation not only provides a model of a current dilemma in medical practice,[3] but also provides an opportunity to consider the nontechnical components of decisions that have individual and societal importance.

1. The Disorder

Neural tube defects are a group of malformations that result from the abnormal closure of the neural tube, which is an early fetal structure. Closure is normally completed by the end of the fourth week of development. About half of the NTDs involve incomplete closure of the neural tube in the developing head region, which leads to anencephaly. This condition is uniformly fatal; the child is either stillborn or dies shortly after birth. The other half of NTDs are various forms of spina bifida (SB), which result from incomplete closure (open SB) or otherwise abnormal development of the spinal cord (closed SB). The degree of impairment associated with spina bifida depends on the location and severity of the lesion. Children may exhibit paralysis of the lower limbs, incontinence, mental retardation, recurrent urinary infections, and hydrocephalus.

NTDs are among the most common serious birth defects in the United States (Goldberg and Oakley, 1979). Although the etiology is unknown, NTDs probably result from inherited predisposition combined with one or more environmental triggers. About 2 to 5% of affected children are born to parents with a family history of NTDs (Gardner, Burton, and Johnson, 1981; Holmes, 1976), but the remaining 95% are born to couples not previously identified as being at risk. The overall incidence per year of neural tube defects in the United States is about 1-2 per 1,000 live births. However, incidence and prevalence vary by ethnic group and geographical location. For example, the incidence of NTDs in Appalachia is well above the overall incidence in the United States, and new cases of NTDs occur about twice as often in whites as in blacks (Greenberg, James, and Oakley, 1983).

2. Screening Procedures

The screening program for neural tube defects potentially involves four procedures: two tests that measure abnormal levels of a fetal protein (alpha-fetoprotein) in the maternal serum; ultrasonography, which permits visualization of the fetus; and amniocentesis, which provides amniotic fluid for further measurements of alpha-fetoprotein and acetylcholinesterase (AChE), an enzyme that is also elevated in the amniotic fluid of affected fetuses. The test series is carried out in the second trimester of pregnancy. Details of each test or procedure are described below.

a. *Measurement of Alpha-fetoprotein.* This test provides the basis for the series of screening procedures outlined above because, if levels of alpha-fetoprotein (AFP) in the maternal serum are within the normal range, no further testing is required. AFP is produced by the fetus in increasing amounts up to 34 weeks of gestation and enters the amniotic fluid. From the fluid, it passes into the maternal serum. The value of the test is that fetuses with neural tube defects have abnormally high levels

11

of AFP in their amniotic fluid and consequently in maternal serum. The test is not definitive, however, since high levels of AFP are found under several conditions, including other malformations, twins (or multiple births), and fetal death. Moreover, since the concentration of AFP in the maternal blood increases up to 34 weeks of gestation, a miscalculation in gestational age could result in an apparently elevated value, i.e., if gestation is believed to be at 16 weeks, but is in fact at 18 weeks, the value would be normal for 18 weeks, but would be falsely high at 16 weeks. There are also problems in providing a definitive value for a "normal" level of MSAFP and, in fact, this value should be determined in each laboratory because standards vary from laboratory to laboratory (see Part II, Section A).

The procedure is simple for the patient and carries no more risk than is usually associated with withdrawal of blood for testing. If the test is positive (i.e., the level of MSAFP is high) and none of the other possible underlying causes can be pinpointed, the mother is referred for a second MSAFP test. If this is also positive without obvious cause the mother may be referred for ultrasonography.

b. *Ultrasonography.* Ultrasonography or ultrasound imaging provides an opportunity for visualization of the fetus, permitting observation of signs of NTDs or other malformations, twin (or multiple) fetuses, or fetal death. It may also be able to indicate miscalculation of the length of gestation since accurate measurement of the size of the fetus is possible. Apart from its ability to rule out other reasons for high levels of MSAFP, ultrasonography can visualize signs of many neural tube defects, although the degree of accuracy depends on the size and location of the defect as well as on the type of equipment and the experience of the operator. The total risks associated with this procedure have not been determined, although no major risks have been identified (Consensus Conference, 1984).

If ultrasonography cannot explain the reason for the high levels of MSAFP, the patient may be offered a final procedure, amniocentesis, to provide amniotic fluid for an additional measurement of AFP and AChE.

c. *Amniocentesis.* Again, this procedure is not specific for diagnosing neural tube defects but is used to provide a sample of amniotic fluid which can then be tested for AFP and for AChE, an enzyme that is also elevated when a neural tube defect is present. During amniocentesis a sample of amniotic fluid is withdrawn from the amniotic sac surrounding the fetus through a needle inserted through the abdominal wall. To be effective for detection of an NTD the procedure is usually performed between the 16th and 20th weeks. If the tests are positive for high levels of AFP and AChE, it is generally considered that an NTD is present. The effectiveness of the test depends on the quality of the sample, however. Contamination with blood will make the result inaccurate. Moreover, the procedure is not without risk because there is invasion of a sterile space, the amniotic sac. Complications include spontaneous abortion, infection, fetomaternal bleeding that increases the fetal death rate, and fetal injury from puncturing the fetus with the needle. Simultaneous monitoring with ultrasonography has decreased these risks. The total risk of fetal death and fetal or maternal morbidity resulting from the procedure, when performed by experienced persons, is in the range of 1% (NICHHD, 1976).

3. Analytic Methods

The analytic methods considered here are distinct but interrelated. Technology assessment produces the basic data from which to build either a cost-effectiveness analysis or a decision analysis. The methodologies for cost-effectiveness analysis and decision analysis share a foundation in probability, modeling techniques, and utility scales.

Technology assessment emphasizes the technical performance of medical tests, where the better choice is the more accurate and safer test. Decision analysis emphasizes the ability to clarify choices in the face of uncertainty or incomplete information. Cost-effectiveness analysis emphasizes the overall efficiency of a medical service for the population where the inefficiencies for individuals carry less weight than efficiencies for the group.

Since protection of well-being, autonomy, and equity are not (and are not meant to be) integral components of the methods but are important to their application, the capability of each analytic method to deal with them is addressed here.

a. *Technology Assessment.* Hamburg (1981) defined the goals of technology assessment as: insuring that technologies with probable benefit and acceptable risk are made available, constraining use of less acceptable technologies, and guiding appropriate use of new and old technologies. He also noted that perhaps only 10 to 20% of all current procedures have been shown to be efficacious in controlled trials and indicated the importance of linking such research to health care innovations. Technology assessment links research and development to prudent application of technologies. A recent comprehensive review of methods, programs, and policies for assessing medical technologies emphasizes the human and economic costs of inadequate evaluation (Institute of Medicine, 1985).

The methods of technology assessment (TA) are used to determine how certain standards have been applied to the tests, procedures, and devices designated for a particular disorder. These standards, efficacy, safety, and effectiveness, are related to the risks and benefits that are presented by the technology. Banta, Behney, and Willems (1981) have defined *efficacy* as the "probability of benefit to individuals in a defined population from a medical technology applied for a given medical problem under ideal conditions of use;" and *safety* as "a judgment of the acceptability of risk in a specified situation," where risk is considered a measure of the "probability and extent of harm to the health of the patient." While efficacy, by this definition, is considered in the context of a controlled research program usually within an academic setting, *effectiveness* is considered as a measure of the benefit from a medical technology under average conditions of use (Banta, Behney, and Willems, 1981). Thus, evaluations of the efficacy, safety, and effectiveness of medical technologies are needed to form an appropriate knowledge base from which the appropriate uses of those technologies may be determined.

Assessing the efficacy and safety of medical technologies used in prenatal diagnosis also helps to evaluate the cost-effectiveness of these technologies and to identify ethical issues associated with their use. For example, if ultrasonography and amniocentesis were shown to lack medical benefit or to be categorically unsafe, the ethical issues regarding the use of those procedures would focus largely upon protecting patients from undue harm.

Technology assessment, therefore, forms a necessary part of a more comprehensive analysis of decision-making in the field of prenatal diagnosis. Assessment of technologies in current use generally begins with a review of the literature. Since published literature may not contain current information and a wide range of methodologies which may not be compatible are used in clinical studies, interpretation of literature reviews is difficult (Wortman and Saxe, 1982; Moses and Brown, 1984). Therefore, TA by literature review can often provide only an estimate of the extent to which efficacy, safety, and effectiveness have been addressed, rather than a definitive evaluation of these issues.

b. *Decision Analysis.* Decision analysis allows the examination of alternative health strategies in a logical manner. It is an explicit process for making choices in situations of uncertainty and in which different opinions and needs must be combined. Decision analysis permits optimal decisions if sufficient data about the problem are available or can be obtained. If sufficient data are not available, the process offers a systematic rational way to examine how different assumptions would affect outcome. Thus, even in the face of great uncertainty decison analysis clarifies thinking and provides the decision maker with insight into the problem (McNeil and Pauker, 1984).

Several elements in decision analysis have been identified. Among them are: structuring the problem so that alternative courses of action can be defined; characterizing the information needed; estimating the probability of chance outcomes; assigning relative value to potential outcomes; choosing a preferred course of action; performing sensitivity analyses with various assumptions; and performing the analyses with the goal of measuring effectiveness as well as the goal of measuring cost. The principles of decision analysis have been reviewed recently by McNeil and Pauker (1984).

For rapidly developing technologies, the information necessary for decision analysis may not be available. However, McNeil and Pauker (1984) point out that DA can clarify the types of information that are needed and the degree of uncertainty that currently affects the analysis. Both the qualitative and quantitative aspects of DA may be useful, even if the quantitative aspects are constrained by limited information.

c. *Cost-Effectiveness Analysis.* Cost-effectiveness analysis (CEA) is used to analyze alternative ways of allocating limited resources (Weinstein et al., 1980). The goal is to find the most effective alternative. Shepard and Thompson (1979) identified five steps in CEA:

• define the scope of the health program and the target population;
• calculate monetary costs of the program;
• determine health effects;
• define and apply decision rules;
• test the strength of the analytic results through sensitivity analyses.

There are several limitations to the accuracy of cost-effectiveness analysis. Definitions of costs and effects will vary depending on the situation under analysis. Quantification of costs and effects is complicated if data are limited. Availability of data also affects the quality of the assumptions that are made, and the quality of those assumptions is a crucial determinant of the validity of the analysis and the results (Sommers, 1984; Stokey and Zeckhauser, 1978). Because of these and other constraints the Office of Technology Assessment observed that CEA is best used in conjunction with other methods of analysis (Office of Technology Assessment, 1980).

In summary, technology assessment identifies what is known about probable performance in best and usual contexts. A decision-analysis can manage uncertainty and identify at least the qualitative elements that bear upon the choices to be made by patients and providers. A cost-effectiveness analysis can estimate the distribution of costs and benefits associated with using the technology in a group or population.

14

C. Results

1. Preliminary Review of Discussion of Ethical Dilemmas in Technical Reports.

A rough indication of the range and nature of references to societal values or ethical issues in publications about prenatal diagnosis was obtained by surveying all of the articles collected in the course of this study.[4] Each article was classified by type, i.e., general review, technology assessment, application of technologies, or primarily ethics. The contents were then rated as containing either *no* discussion related to values or ethical issues, *some* discussion, or *major* discussion (Table 1).

We observed that the majority of this selected literature on prenatal diagnosis contained only some reference (32%) or no reference (45%) to such issues. The articles rated as containing "some" reference generally raised ethical questions but did not discuss them. Typically, these articles either included mention of "nonmedical" factors (financial costs, psychological benefits, public attitudes) in the application of prenatal diagnostic technologies or referred to a specific moral conflict that might arise through the application of these technologies. The majority of the articles with no reference to societal or ethical concerns were clinically-oriented empirical studies or case reports. The remaining 23% of the articles were concerned primarily with ethical, legal or public policy matters. For example, in a recent paper, Leaf (1984) presents the dilemma faced by physicians today who can no longer consider only the best interests of the individual patient, but must be concerned with cost of medical services and priorities for allocation of resources. The paper makes suggestions for steps that the medical profession together with the public might take to reduce areas of conflict. The first suggestion is to assess new technologies much more carefully so that both benefits and costs can be considered before introducing them into practice.

Table 1
Discussion of values or ethics in 143 recent publications in the field of prenatal diagnosis

	Degree of discussion		
Type of Article	None	Some	Major
Review (24%)	11	18	5
Technology assessment (11%)	11	4	0
Application (49%)	43	22	6
Ethics (16%)	0	2	21
Total	65 (45%)	46 (32%)	32 (23%)

Similarly, Holtzman (1984) examines issues in TA for prenatal diagnosis of phenylketonuria with the objective of reducing ignorance before technologies are introduced into practice. Both authors address the need to discuss relevant ethical issues. They offer discussion on TA and costs that are related to ethical concerns, but treat these concerns in a general fashion.

In summary, papers that deal with technical or analytical techniques do not deal with ethical concerns to any extent, and even those papers that are purported to discuss ethical issues tend to skirt them. To be sure, this sample of papers is by no means definitive, but this review emphasizes the need for explicit and informed consideration of ethical concerns that are immediately relevant. A step in this direction was taken by the Committee for Evaluating Medical Technologies in Clinical Use whose recent book (Institute of Medicine, 1985) discusses social and ethical issues in technology assessment.

We next examined how the three analytic techniques selected (technology assessment, decision analysis, and cost-effectiveness analysis) applied to prenatal detection of neural tube defects do or do not help in making decisions that uphold the three ethical principles of well-being, autonomy, and equity previously described. The results of the analytic studies are summarized first (and detailed in Part II), followed by a discussion that interprets the results in the context of the ethical principles. The summaries are principally excerpts from the analyses.

2. Technology Assessment by Literature Review (Kiely and Meister)

Part II, Section A[5] illustrates a literature-based technology assessment. This analysis was designed to establish how well the literature addresses the major components of technology assessment (safety, efficacy, effectiveness), rather than to assess directly those attributes in NTD screening.

The authors propose that assessing the technologies used in screening for neural tube defects should cover two levels of analysis: (1) the individual technologies; and (2) the complete screening sequence. They found that the published reports emphasize studies of the individual technologies. The papers that discuss pilot screening programs analyze the screening sequence, but emphasize diagnostic outcomes. The focus takes little account of factors such as interactions between tests, a broad range of patient outcomes, and the clinical course of patients who did not follow the usual screening protocol. In general, technology assessment of NTD screening provides uneven information. Especially compelling gaps in knowledge are identified by the authors and are listed below.

MSAFP. New mathematical models for interpreting maternal serum alpha-fetoprotein values make use of maternal factors, such as weight and medical history, and fetal factors, such as gestational age. In terms of the effectiveness of MSAFP, are these data likely to be available? In terms of efficacy, are these models equally useful for all forms of MSAFP calibration?

Pilot studies of NTD screening indicate that a significant number of women do not participate in MSAFP screening. Should the physician include a discussion of MSAFP as part of prenatal care? What are choices about screening based on? Who makes these choices, why are they made, and what happens to the pregnancies of women who do not participate in the screening?

Ultrasonography. The report of the NIH Consensus Conference on Diagnostic Ultrasound Imaging in Pregnancy pointed out that it is essential to continue to evaluate the safety of this procedure. The report also raised issues regarding standards for equipment and operator training. Those issues are also pertinent to the assessment of efficacy and effectiveness.

The appropriate use of ultrasonographic findings is currently undetermined. Reports indicate that confidence in the findings varies among clinicians, which leaves some uncertainty about the diagnostic impact of ultrasonography. Does (and should) ultrasonography replace other tests such as amniocentesis? If so, under what conditions?

Amniocentesis for measurement of AFP and AChE. Recent findings suggest methods for reducing complications of amniocentesis. Are there other factors, such as anxiety or stress, which affect the probability of untoward effects?

The accuracy of amniotic fluid AFP measurement depends on the quality of the sample of amniotic fluid. Even assuming high quality samples, the methods for calibrating the test results and establishing cutoffs for abnormal values present the same problems found in MSAFP testing. Although the literature illustrates the role of AChE in improving diagnostic accuracy, this test was not included in the pilot NTD screening programs included in this review. Would the improved diagnostic power be seen in large-scale applications?

Should these tests be used as the final step in testing, or should ultrasonography become the next step? Kiely and Meister found little analysis of the relative costs and benefits to be expected if ultrasonography were used to confirm AFP and AChE findings.

The overall screening protocol. They also found little discussion or analysis of the availability of the screening tests. There was even less discussion of specific issues, such as access to the most appropriate equipment and operators, supportive services, and the resources that make a range of parental choices truly possible.

Kiely and Meister also found little discussion of the effects of screening on two groups: women who do not follow the usual screening protocol, and the fetus.

In one of the pilot studies, diagnostic accuracy of the screening protocol was enhanced by the use of a coordinated system of expert obstetricians, clinical geneticists, experienced laboratory staff, and ultrasonographers (Milunsky and Alpert, 1984). However, the authors found little analysis of how these factors should be integrated when considering the value of NTD screening for a population.

Finally, Kiely and Meister found no studies that describe a broad range of costs and benefits to pregnant women undergoing NTD screening, with psychological dimensions being most neglected.

Technology assessment is used most frequently to examine and refine tests and laboratory procedures. In that case, the standards of efficacy, effectiveness, and safety are goals to be achieved. Here, the authors used the standards as the benchmarks of well-balanced and comprehensive knowledge. They propose that this approach to technology assessment offers a unique opportunity to see the field as a whole. The findings are important because they describe the quality of knowledge about the technologies. For example, if the literature about the technologies used in prenatal NTD screening fully addressed the standards of efficacy, effectiveness, and safety, it would provide a sound basis for determining how best to use the technologies. When the basis is not as sound, it is important to know where the gaps are. This kind of information is especially useful to health care professionals and state and federal policymakers responsible for determining the testing protocols that should be made available to all pregnant women.

The major conclusion of the literature review on technology assessment in Part

17

II, Section A is that technology assessment through literature review cannot answer all of the questions about applications of medical technology, but the questions that are answered and the gaps in knowledge that are identified provide valuable information for planning and for research.

3. Decision Analysis (McNeil and Pauker)

Section II, Part B[6] examines how decision analysis could be applied to one of the screening procedures used in prenatal screening for neural tube defects. In particular, the authors were concerned with determining to what extent the process of decision analysis can contribute to decisions about appropriate use of prenatal diagnostic technologies. Decision analysis is currently being used increasingly in health-related analyses as it is concerned with quantifying clinical issues that are associated with uncertainty (McNeil and Pauker, 1984). The authors chose second trimester obstetrical ultrasonographic screening for analysis because it is not only part of the overall screening procedure for neural tube defects, but it can be used to detect a variety of fetal disorders. In this respect, decisions regarding its most effective use assume greater importance; moreover, use of ultrasonography is rapidly becoming more widespread, its accuracy is variable, and its long term effects are uncertain (Department of Health and Human Services, 1984).

Decision analysis is an approach, actually a set of modeling techniques, that provides insight into the tradeoffs inherent in the decision at hand. Decision analysis is a formal and explicit way of answering such questions as "What is the most cost-effective approach to screening small children for lead poisoning?" Or, "What is the extra cost per extra quality-adjusted life-year gained from introducing diagnostic test 'X' or treatment 'Y'?"

Use of decision analysis to help determine the value of a screening program for neural tube defects first requires the creation of a model giving the alternatives. Figure 2 illustrates one model for this purpose (Pauker, Pauker, and McNeil, 1981). In this diagram, points of decision ("decision nodes") are depicted by squares, whereas outcomes occurring by chance ("chance nodes") are depicted by circles.

According to this tree the alternatives involve a decision between screening (upper branch) and no screening (lower branch). If screening is undertaken and is normal, the fetus is presumed to be at low risk for having an NTD. If the screening is abnormal, it is repeated and if the second test is also abnormal, ultrasonography is recommended. The second decision node of the upper branch indicates that the patient can either accept or refuse ultrasonography. In the former case, the examination will indicate an explanation for the abnormal AFP level (e.g., by showing twins), will show the presence of an NTD, or will not give a satisfactory explanation for the abnormal AFP. These latter two alternatives are associated with choices on the part of the patient, as shown in the figure. As the reader follows the consequences resulting from each of these decisions, he or she will always end at a common subtree, shown as a diamond, or at an induced interruption of pregnancy, or at a miscarriage.

These "outcome nodes" at eight points of the "screen" strategy and at one point of the "no screen" strategy all have the same structure shown at the bottom of the figure. As a result of the interventions up to this point in the tree a patient can either miscarry or proceed through a pregnancy and have a child with or without an NTD. The chances of these outcomes differ at various points in the decision tree depending upon the sequence of diagnostic data leading to that point. For example, the like-

Figure 2
Decision Tree for Prenatal NTD Screening

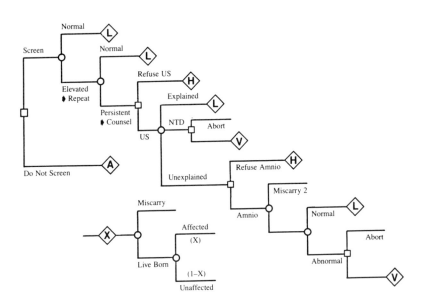

Decision tree for the alpha-fetoprotein decision. The main tree is shown in the top part of the figure; the subtree with X in the diamond denotes the outcomes of pregnancy and is depicted in the lower portion of the figure. Each reference to the subtree is denoted by a diamond. The letter within the diamond refers to the risk of an affected fetus: A for average risk, L for lower than average risk, H for high risk, and V for very high risk. These risks were calculated using Bayes rule (Weinstein et. al., 1980) NTD = neural tube defect; AMNIO = amniocentesis; ABORT = elective abortion; MISCARRY 2 = miscarriage secondary to amniocentesis.

Reproduced with permission from *Ann Rev Public Health* 1984, 5:141.

lihood would be high (H) after two abnormal AFP determinations not explained by another cause, but low (L) after a single normal serum test.

McNeil and Pauker point out that in order to determine the relative values of the "screen" and "no screen" strategies in the above decision tree *probability* estimates must be attached at each of the chance nodes. For example, "how often will ultrasonography reveal an error in the estimated gestational age or the presence of twins in women with two elevated AFP levels?" "What is the excess miscarriage rate for women having second trimester amniocentesis?" It is also necessary in this analysis to attach values or *utilities* to the four possible outcomes occurring in this situation: parents' attitudes towards an accidental miscarriage resulting from amniocentesis; their attitudes towards an elective abortion; and their attitudes towards the birth of a child affected with a neural tube defect. The birth of a healthy child is assumed to be the best outcome. The third step in the process involves serial multiplications of probabilities times utilities so that the expected utility of the two strategies can be compared.

At least conceptually, probabilistic data can be obtained in a straightforward manner. For the AFP problem, data from Great Britain and U.S. studies are applicable. They would answer the above questions as follows: 50% of women will have an explanation for two abnormal AFP levels. The excess miscarriage rate from amniocentesis is probably about 0.5%.

Utility data, on the other hand, are more difficult to obtain and must nearly always be acquired as part of the analysis in question. There are no "utility data banks" to help the analyst. Utility assessments require that attitudes for the conditions under study be placed on a scale from zero to 100, in this case zero implying the birth of a normal child and 100 the birth of a child with a neural tube defect. The value of another outcome, say an abortion, is obtained by responses to questions of the form "At what chance of a pregnancy's producing a severely deformed child would you prefer elective abortion to the risk of having a live-born child affected with a neural tube defect?" The minimum chance at which they would still prefer abortion is used as a measure of the burden of abortion relative to the burden of an affected child. An analogous question is required to assess the burden of a miscarriage introduced by amniocentesis. An article by Christensen-Szalanski (1984) may be of interest to readers concerned about the stability of such utility assessments over time.

The authors use fixed values of each of the probabilities and utilities to give expected utilities for the "screen" and "no screen" strategies. In this case, the decision problem was formulated for society and does not address the issue for an individual patient. Thus, the analysis becomes more complex and varies with the distribution of values in the society for the possible outcomes (miscarriage, abortion, child with NTD). This distribution influences the extent to which the population being considered would benefit by having the serum screen introduced so that subsequent options are possible. The reader is referred to the original article (Pauker, Pauker, and McNeil, 1981) for a further discussion of the details of this analysis.

A similar analysis was done for the value of ultrasonographic examinations for screening in the second trimester of pregnancy (see Section II, Part B). The results can be summarized as follows. With routine screening for any of the possible abnormalities, the major effects of ultrasonography are the prevention of the birth of some defective fetuses and the movement of the monetary costs of intervention from the perinatal to the prenatal period. Costs would be reduced because selective interruption of pregnancy is less expensive than treatment (Lau and Pauker, 1984).

Even more interesting results occur when maternal serum AFP screening and a routine second trimester ultrasonographic examination are viewed together (Lau and Pauker, 1984). If the maternal serum AFP is *not* elevated, then the chance of an NTD (the most common type of anomaly detected by ultrasonographic screening) is lowered sufficiently to make screening no longer cost-effective.

Although decision analyses can be time-consuming and frustrating because of difficulties in obtaining reliable data, the authors find that use of this technique in the medical field appears to be increasing. Recently, as part of several Consensus Development Conferences sponsored by the NIH, decision analyses have been done simultaneously with the more conventional "expert consensus" approach. This trend may well continue and extend to other organizations. Because of society's current concern with its limited resources for health, it will become increasingly important for us to answer a series of "what if" questions in a timely fashion. Advances in molecular genetics suggest that decisions involving prenatal diagnosis and therapy *in utero* may benefit from this technique.

4. Cost-effectiveness Analysis (Meister, Shepard, and Zeckhauser)

Part II, Section C[7] illustrates how cost-effectiveness analysis can be applied to a clinical problem. The methodology clarifies complex clinical issues, makes underlying values explicit, and systematically tests critical variables. On the other hand, the validity of the analysis depends on either having appropriate data or the ability to make assumptions. Performing the analysis on a hypothetical cohort makes the analysis possible, but it also limits its usefulness for the clinician who must resolve these same questions with individual patients.

The authors defined a hypothetical cohort of one million pregnant women who receive prenatal care at 16 weeks. To obtain results relevant to most of the pregnant women in the population, the authors assumed that the members of the cohort had no family history of NTD. Meister et al. also assumed that all women consented to the initial screening procedure, although total consent was not found in pilot programs. A sensitivity analysis of this assumption would be useful, but to simplify a complex presentation, the authors did not include it here.

Next, the authors examined four published reports of womens' participation in NTD screening programs. Macri et al. (1979a and b) and Gardner, Burton, and Johnson (1981) each screened 3,500 to 5,000 pregnancies. Nelson (1983) reported on NTD screening among 14,561 women. All four reports were used to estimate the probable participation patterns of the hypothetical cohort. For example, some women who have an abnormal test result will decline further testing. The reports were also used to calculate the proportion of those declining and where data were available, the percentage of women who would experience spontaneous fetal death before the next test.

This analysis examined how a prenatal screening program for NTDs would contribute to improving the chances of acting in accordance with participants' personal values and preferences.

One innovation by the authors is a recognition that the effects of a testing program will differ radically between two groups: women who would choose to abort an affected fetus and women who would choose to continue the pregnancy and prepare. Preparation for the birth of a baby with a neural tube defect is important to the outcome for that child. Optimal therapy of an NTD with meningomyelocele includes surgery to close the skin defect. To prevent meningeal infection, the surgery should be done within 48 hours of birth. Careful monitoring for development of hydrocephalus, which also must be treated surgically, is essential. Because of the neurosurgical, urinary and orthopedic aspects of this condition, children do much better if cared for by a multidisciplinary clinical group. Thus, when an NTD is diagnosed prenatally, preparation for delivery in a hospital equipped to deal promptly and expertly with the condition can influence the degree of permanent impairment. Plans for the care of the infant and interventions to support psychological adjustment of the mother and family are also important.

The author's approach to the analysis employs separate utility scales for the two groups of women. They leave the decision whether to abort or prepare to individuals and assess the costs and benefits that follow from their choices. Without introducing further value judgments, there is no valid way to combine results for these two groups into a single cost-effectiveness assessment.

Meister, Shepard, and Zeckhauser used two utility scales: one for women who would choose abortion and one for women who would choose to prepare for the birth of an affected child. The authors point out that it is especially difficult to construct utility scales when the analysis includes multiple outcomes, because the scale must place a number of treatments and outcomes in some sort of order. Errors (false positives and false negatives) occur in screening, and therefore, the utility scales are actually disutility or loss scales. The scales do not represent the views of any individual but rather, estimates of how the two groups of women might rank order the losses associated with diagnostic errors. The authors' scales use "equivalent losses avoided" (ELA) as the unit of measurement, and that unit is the failure to diagnose one case of spina bifida. The two scales weigh the gains from identifying spina bifida and anencephaly against the losses from misdiagnosing unaffected fetuses.

The basic analysis uses the 95th percentile as the cutoff between normal and elevated MSAFP. The sensitivity analysis uses the 99th percentile. The outcomes of the basic analysis of the screening program in the hypothetical cohort are as follows: 925 women are diagnosed as having an NTD-affected fetus. This diagnosis is correct for 90 percent of the women; 412 of 699 fetuses with anencephaly and 424 of 819 fetuses with spina bifida are identified. Unavoidably, 89 unaffected fetuses (about 1 in 11,000) are misdiagnosed as abnormal after screening is completed. Screening leaves 7,693 women with incorrect positive findings based on incomplete screening. There are 296 women with incomplete screening who have correct, negative findings. The program was calculated to cost about $39 per participant, more than half of which is due to the first screening test. In California, a statewide MSAFP program was signed into law on April 7, 1986. According to the May 9, 1986 *American Medical News*, the annual cost of caring for a child with a NTD is estimated to be from $40,000 to $50,000. The basis for the estimate was not given.

Is this screening program worthwhile for the participants? The authors point out that in a program that emphasizes free choice, participants can always decide to ignore admittedly imperfect tests. Provided participants are fully informed and free to respond to information as they see best, any screening program must be beneficial or neutral on average *to them*. If the inconvenience and the medical and financial costs to them were sufficient, not a likely problem with prenatal NTD screening, they might choose not to participate. Alternative loss functions could also be considered. For utility scales that assign a sufficiently heavy penalty to misclassifying a normal fetus, for example, prenatal screening for NTDs would be disadvantageous to a pregnant woman.

The authors observed that limitations on available data preclude a comprehensive numerical result. The results described here depend on both uncertain data and assumptions and because of their inherent limitations should be interpreted with care. According to Meister et al., the study cannot provide answers to a number of important questions regarding the efficacy of NTD screening for the pregnant population, but was successful in applying cost-effectiveness analysis to a complex clinical issue. It yields important conclusions on some issues and identifies the critical inputs required to reach conclusions on other issues.

To summarize the numerical results, for women who would prepare, the cost per equivalent losses avoided (ELA) ranges from $87,000 to $90,000 depending on the cutoff for the first test. Such a program may well be justified in terms of cost, depending on the valuation of the medical gains and the cost savings that may come from preparation and early medical intervention. Now that NTD screening programs are actually being used, research on the magnitude of these benefits becomes a priority issue.

For women who would abort and who accept the fact that testing will occasionally misdiagnose an unaffected pregnancy, this screening program not only increases their welfare, but saves economic resources. The cost per ELA ranges from $86,000 to $92,000, depending on the cutoff used in the first test. These costs seem likely to be outweighed by savings in lifetime costs of caretaking and medical treatment.

The authors' intent was to demonstrate that cost-effectiveness analysis provides a useful framework for organizing the information about preferences, probabilities, and costs needed to evaluate a screening program and to describe the performance of the NTD test protocol. The analysis developed an output measure, *dollar cost per ELA*, that assessed effectiveness as loss from optimal performance. The authors suggest that this measure should serve as a useful guidepost for evaluating other medical interventions as well as NTD screening. For preparers, additional data—notably the implications of preparation for lifetime medical costs of a child with spina bifida—and value judgments are required to determine whether the screening program is worthwhile. For aborters, the screening program is worthwhile on both criteria employed: cost savings and the women's self-assessed welfare.

In summary, the example of prenatal screening for neural tube defects shows that cost-effectiveness analysis can provide a framework for incorporating new information as it becomes available, and help to clarify a decision problem. In this way, it can promote decisions based on the most recent scientific information, taking into account both the pitfalls and the advantages of the analytic method.

D. Discussion

In the example of NTD screening, we found that each analytic method addressed only some facet of each ethical principle or societal value (Table 2). Even though each value is addressed to some extent by conducting all three analyses, the results do not provide a comprehensive basis for ensuring ethical decision-making.

Table 2

Links between analytic findings and societal values in screening for neural tube defects

	Well-being	Autonomy	Equity
Results of technology assessment	X	X	
Results of decision analysis	X	X	
Results of cost-effectiveness analysis	X		X

The TA review identified unanswered questions in the field. Research to answer these questions would give information on the efficacy, safety, and effectiveness of the technologies. By evaluating these factors, particularly safety, TA aids in upholding the principle of well-being by avoiding the possible harm from premature application of new techniques.

TA results indicated a wide range of both risks and benefits in screening for NTDs. This kind of information is especially important to patients and providers

23

since it gives both groups the data from which to formulate choices. In this way TA identified some implications for autonomy. Nevertheless, TA did not address the role of values in individual choices; it only clarified the risks and benefits that would follow from particular choices. TA did not provide insight into how technologies can be applied fairly or equally, and therefore did not address equity.

Decision analysis was predicated upon identifying all possible outcomes of clinical events and choices. In the instances where data were adequate, the probability of each outcome was established. DA then addressed well-being because it quantified the potential for harm or benefit to the patient. The degree to which DA makes this contribution is determined jointly by the available knowledge, validity of assumptions, and the quality of the analysis.

DA emphasized the role and effect of freedom of choice, dominant themes in autonomy. This emphasis is particularly evident in the utilities that are assigned to clinical outcomes. For example, Pauker, Pauker, and McNeil (1981) describe a detailed methodology for representing prospective parents' relative values for spontaneous fetal death, birth of an NTD-affected child, and elective termination of pregnancy. This approach yields utility scales that are a quantification of individual values. If utility scales accurately represent both the range and the rank order of these values, they contribute to understanding the principle of autonomy.

This same process could be applied to a DA of a provider's choices and contribute to understanding the issues related to respecting the values of health care providers as well.

By its nature, decision analysis emphasizes individual values and decision-making, rather than costs. Since both fairness and equality deal with costs and values, decision analysis does not contribute directly to understanding equity in distribution of the benefits of prenatal diagnosis of NTDs.

Cost-effectiveness analysis addresses well-being in the same way as decision analysis because it includes individual values and decision-making. It does not address autonomy, however, because it focuses only on costs and effects for the group rather than the individual. For this reason, cost-effectiveness analysis does address one facet of equity. It clearly describes how costs, risks, and effects are distributed in a group, but it does not address how they should be distributed and thus, addresses equality but not fairness.

CEA allows us to identify risk of diagnostic errors at each step of the screening program. Therefore, it identifies the parts of the screening process that result in certain groups bearing higher risks than others, which is an important issue in terms of equity. Cost-effectiveness analysis identifies the distribution of risk and contributes to an understanding of how equally that risk is shared and by which groups. We cannot, however, go further and consider the *fairness* of the distribution. An analysis of who "should" bear risk requires different information.

E. Conclusion

We tested three quantitative methods that are commonly used in decision-making (TA, DA, and CEA) and conclude that whereas each method has something specific to offer, no single analytic tool is able to point to the decisions about prenatal diagnosis of NTDs that are in full consonance with our society's desired values.

All three methods produced information that can clarify choices about using the technologies, but the validity, completeness, and timeliness of the methods varied. The underlying assumptions, scope of analysis, and degree of attention to individual decision-making affect the results of CEA. The analytic results of TA are affected by the rigor of the analysis and available data. The results of DA depend on the validity of the assumptions and of the analytic model. All of the analyses depend on accurate data. For prenatal diagnosis, the data must also be timely. The categories of congenital disorders described earlier help to clarify how options change as the availability of data increases. In fields with rapid development, such as prenatal diagnosis, the analyses will need to be repeated as new information is generated.

Insufficient information often leads to societal dilemmas. In the case of NTDs, a far from perfect test and lack of early prenatal care for all pregnant women results in serious problems of, for example, resource allocation for prenatal diagnosis. Nevertheless, dilemmas also point to what research is urgently needed: in development of a specific and accurate prenatal test for NTDs on the one hand and in delivery of health services on the other. The ultimate goals of an inexpensive, "perfect" test and full, early prenatal care would eliminate some dilemmas. Even then, dilemmas related to other policies and problems would remain. Coverage of payment for selective interruption of pregnancy and access to special services are two critical examples.

Despite the problems of validity, completeness, and timeliness illustrated in the analyses described in Part II of this report, these three analyses are being used with rapidly increasing frequency in the medical field. CEA in particular is a seductive tool for decisions about allocation of resources in public health. In the face of limited resources coupled with rapidly expanding and often costly technical capabilities for prenatal diagnosis (not matched by rapid improvements in treatment), ethical and societal problems with no obvious solutions abound.

We tried to assess in a preliminary way how three analytic tools could help to preserve the ethical principles for health care outlined by the President's Commission for the Study of Ethical Problems in Medicine and Biomedical and Behavioral Research. Overall, it seems that each of the analytic methods contributes to upholding aspects of one or two of the bioethical principles. However, none of the analytic methods illuminates all aspects of any ethical issue, nor was any one designed to do so. Even taken together, the analytic results fall short of clarifying the meaning of all of the ethical issues that are central to making the best decisions about application of prenatal diagnostic technologies.

Even so, the analyses provide a valuable contribution. When the results do address an issue, both the results and the analysis that produced them are clearly evident. This clarity sharpens thinking, enhances evaluation and critique, and encourages advances in understanding the field.

Clearly, several methods used in combination would be preferable to any method used alone, and explicit consideration of ethical issues should be included in technical assessments. Collaboration among health care providers, other technical experts, and those knowledgeable about ethics and societal values should be strongly encouraged. With changing circumstances, as illustrated by the four categories of disorders cited earlier, policy options for a particular condition will change as will the emphasis placed on one or the other of the ethical principles discussed here (Veatch, 1984). Although historically our society has placed great value on freedom of choice, severely constrained fiscal resources may make it necessary to emphasize fairness to a greater extent than before. Any consideration of social benefits and costs of a technology should include consideration of alternative uses of the money (Institute of Medicine, 1985), and, in the allocation of resources for research, the

25

large gap between prenatal diagnostic and treatment capabilities. According to Edmund Pellegrino, "Health policies are rarely derived from explicit and systematic analysis of the moral values that shape them. However, once framed, a health policy unerringly reveals the values that drive a society; and these cannot escape examination retrospectively" (Pellegrino, 1985). These points illustrate why discussions of ethics and values should play a major role in decision-making on an ongoing basis.

As the Institute of Medicine report (1985) points out, social, ethical, and legal questions raised by the use of technologies in clinical practice can be systematically identified and evaluated (even if not quantified) and lead to better decisions. In contrast, as illustrated here, technology assessments, cost-effectiveness studies, and other analyses appear to be objective because they are quantitative; but, in fact, selected data underlie the assumptions for the quantitative analyses. Selection of data is influenced in turn by subjective and value judgements that are submerged and lost in the numbers. Thus, the results of these "objective" analyses in fact depend on the personal values of the analyst and on available data.

Whatever the future holds in the field of prenatal diagnosis, rather than relying on the developers and proponents of technologies or on economic pressures alone, it is better to consider the societal aspects of the decisions that will have to be made seriously, early on, and from a truly multidisciplinary perspective. Policy formulation in this and other rapidly advancing fields takes place at the interface of facts and values. At the very least, decisions should be made in full awareness of this, changed in timely fashion as evidence changes, and with full participation by those whose interests are clinical or technical as well as those who are concerned with upholding our society's vaues. Continued amplification and refinement of analytic methods such as those described here are to be supported and encouraged because thoughtful and well reasoned analyses clarify thinking and point to gaps in knowledge that need to be filled. In spite of current limitations, use of several technical analyses in concert, coupled with explicit and systematic analysis of pertinent societal and ethical values, will have the best chance of providing everyone with technically optimal and humane prenatal diagnostic care.

F. Footnotes

[1]The term congenital disorders is used here to refer to the entire range of disorders, genetic and nongenetic, present at birth (Emery and Rimoin, 1983).

[2]Under the auspices of the Division of Health Policy Research and Education, Harvard University. The project was sponsored by two of the Division's Working Groups: Early Life and Adolescent Health Policy (Julius B. Richmond, M.D., Chair) and Disease Prevention and Health Promotion (Alexander Leaf, M.D., Chair), and supported by a grant from the Robert Wood Johnson Foundation. The project study group is listed in Appendix 2 and the Working Group rosters are Appendix 3a and 3b. We extend special thanks to Fredric Frigoletto, Jr., M.D. for his invaluable and generous contributions.

[3]For example, as of May 1986, as indicated in a letter to members, the American Society of Human Genetics (ASHG) could not agree on a statement of policy and practice on maternal serum alpha-fetoprotein screening. Note added in proof: The ASHG issued a policy statement on MSAFP screening "intended as suggestions only" on November 2, 1986.

[4]We thank Stephen Buka for his contributions to the survey and the discussion of ethical issues.

[5]"Literature on prenatal screening for neural tube defects: standards of technology assessment," Mary L. Kiely, Ph.D. and Susan B. Meister, Ph.D., R.N. (Review ended in 1984.)

[6]"Prenatal screening for neural tube defects: use of decision analysis," Barbara McNeil, M.D., Ph.D. and Stephen G. Pauker, M.D.

[7]"Cost-effectiveness of prenatal screening for neural tube defects," Susan B. Meister, Ph.D., R.N., Donald Shepard, Ph.D., and Richard Zeckhauser, Ph.D.

G. References

Adams, M.M., Oakley, G.P., and Marks, J.S. Maternal age and births in the 1980s. *Journal of the American Medical Association*, 1982, *247*, 493-494.

American College of Obstetricians and Gynecologists. Professional liability alert for MSAFP. Special notice to ACOG Fellows from the Law Department of ACOG, May 1985.

Banta, H.D., Behney, C.J., and Willems, J.S. *Toward rational technology in medicine*, New York: Springer Publishing Company, 1981.

Beauchamp, T.L. Ethical theory and bioethics. In *Contemporary issues in bioethics*.T. Beauchamp and L. Walters (Eds.), California: Wadsworth Publishing Co., 2nd edition, 1982.

Christensen-Szalanski, J.J. Discount functions and the measurement of patients' values: Women's decisions during childbirth. *Medical Decision Making*, 1984, *4*, 47-58.

Consensus Conference. The use of diagnostic ultrasound imaging during pregnancy. *Journal of the American Medical Association*, 1984, *252*, 669-672.

Cowart, V. First-trimester prenatal diagnostic method becoming available in U.S. *Journal of the American Medical Association*, 1983, *250*, 1249-1250.

Cuckle, A.E.H. and Wald, N.J. Maternal serum alpha-fetoprotein measurement: A screening test for Down Syndrome. *Lancet*, 1984, *1*, 926-932.

Department of Health and Human Service. *Diagnostic ultrasound imaging in pregnancy: Report of a consensus conference*. Washington: Superintendent of Documents, 1984. (NIH Publication No. 84-667.)

Emery, A.E.H. and Rimoin, D.L. *Principles and practice of medical genetics*. New York: Churchill Livingstone Inc., 1983.

Gardner S., Burton, B.K., and Johnson, A.M. Maternal serum alpha-fetoprotein screening: A report of the Forsyth County Project. *American Journal of Obstetrics and Gynecology*, 1981, *140*, 250-253.

Goldberg, M.F. and Oakley, G.P. Prenatal screening for anencephaly-spina bifida: Some epidemiological projections for a national program. In I.H. Porter and E.B. Hook (Eds.), *Service and education in medical genetics*. New York: Academic Press, 1979.

Greenberg, F., James, L.M., and Oakley, G.P. Estimates of birth prevalence rates of Spina Bifida in the United States from computer-generated maps. *American Journal of Obstetrics and Gynecology*, 1983, *145*, 570-573.

Gusella, J.F., Wexler, N.S., Conneally, P.M., et al. A polymorphic DNA marker genetically linked to Huntington's Disease. *Nature*, 1983, *306*, 234-238.

Hamburg, D.A. Toward more judicious use of biomedical technology in health care. In *Evaluating medical technologies in clinical use* (IOM Publ. No. 81-004). Washington, D.C.: National Academy Press, 1981.

Hobbins, J.C., Venus, I., Tortora, M., Mayden, K., and Mahoney, M.J. Stage II ultrasound examination for the diagnosis of fetal abnormalities with elevated amniotic fluid alpha-fetoprotein concentrations. *American Journal of Obstetrics and Gynecology*, 1982, *142*, 1026-1029.

Holmes, L.B., Driscoll, S.G., and Atkins, L. Etiologic heterogeneity of neural tube defects. *New England Journal of Medicine*, 1976, *294*, 365-369.

Holtzmann, N.A. Ethical issues in the prenatal diagnosis of phenylketonuria. *Pediatrics* 1984, *74*, 424-427.

Hook, E.B., Schreinemachers, D.M., and Cross, P.K. Use of prenatal cytogenetic diagnosis in New York state. *New England Journal of Medicine*, 1981, *305*, 1410-1413.

Institute of Medicine. Committee for evaluating medical technologies in clinical use. *Assessing medical technology*. Washington, D.C.: National Academy Press, 1985.

Lappe, M. Predictive power of the new genetics. *The Hastings Center Report*, 1984, *14*, 18-21.

Lau, J. and Pauker, S.G. The use of diagnostic ultrasound imaging in pregnancy. NIH Consensus Development Conference Decision Analysis Project. Feb. 6-8, 1984, Bethesda, Md.

Leaf, A. The doctor's dilemma—and society's too. *New England Journal of Medicine*, 1984, *310*, 718-721.

Lewin, R. Shifting sentiments over sequencing the human genome. *Science*, 1986, *233*, 620-621.

Macri, J.N., Haddow, J.E., and Weiss, R.R. Screening for neural tube defects in the United States. *American Journal Obstetrics and Gynecology*, 1979a, *133*, 119-125.

Macri, J.N., Weiss, R.R., and Libster, B. Maternal serum alpha-fetoprotein screening for neural tube defects: Structure and organization. In Porter, I.H., and Hook, E.B. (Eds.) *Service and education in medical genetics*. New York: Academic Press, 1979b.

McKusick, V.A. *Mendelian inheritance in man*. (6th ed.) Baltimore: Johns Hopkins University Press, 1983.

McNeil, B.J. and Pauker, S.G. Decision analysis for public health: Principles and illustrations. *Annual Review of Public Health*, 1984, *5*, 135-161.

Milunsky, A. and Alpert, E. Results and benefits of a maternal serum alpha-fetoprotein screening program. *Journal of the American Medical Association*, 1984, *252*, 1438-1442.

Modell, B. Chorionic villus sampling: Evaluating safety and efficacy. *Lancet*, 1985, *1*, 737-740.

Moses, L.E. and Brown, B.W., Jr. Experiences with evaluating the safety and efficacy of medical technologies. *Annual Review of Public Health*, 1984, *5*, 267-292.

Murray, R.F., Chamberlain, N., Fletcher, J., Hopkins, E., Jackson, R., King, P.A., and Powledge, T.M. Special considerations for minority participation in prenatal diagnosis. *Journal of the American Medical Association*, 1980, *243*, 1254-1256.

National Academy of Sciences. *Genetic screening: Programs, principles, and research.* Washington, D.C.: National Academy of Sciences, 1975.

National Institute of Child Health and Human Development. National Registry for Amniocentesis Study Group. Midtrimester amniocentesis for prenatal diagnosis: safety and accuracy. *Journal of the American Medical Association*, 1976, *236*, 1471-1476.

Nelson, L.H. Neural tube defects. Paper presented at the 1983 American Institute of Ultrasound in Medicine/Society of Diagnostic Medical Sonographers Annual Convention. New York, New York. October, 1983.

Office of Technology Assessment. *The implications of cost-effectiveness analysis of medical technology*. Washington, D.C.: U.S. Government Printing Office, 1980.

Pauker, S.G., Pauker, S.P., and McNeil, B.J. The effect of private attitudes on public policy: Prenatal screening for neural tube defects as a prototype. *Medical Decision Making*, 1981, *1*, 103-114.

Pellegrino. E. *Health policy: Ethics and human values. (An international dialogue)*. Highlights of the Athens Conference. Council for International Organizations of Medical Sciences ISBN 9290360216 Switzerland, 1985.

Powledge, T.M. and Fletcher, J. Guidelines for the ethical, social and legal issues in prenatal diagnosis. *New England Journal of Medicine*, 1979, *300*, 168-172.

President's Commission for the Study of Ethical Problems in Medicine and Biomedical and Behavioral Research. *Summing up: Final report on studies of the ethical and legal problems in medicine and biomedical and behavioral research*. Washington, D.C.: U.S. Government Printing Office, March, 1983. #040-000-00475-1.

Richmond, J.B. and Holtzman, N.A. Prevention of chronic illness in children: Genetic strategies. In Perrin, J.M. and Shayne, M.W. (Eds.) *Public policies affecting chronically-ill children and their families*. San Francisco: Jossey-Bass, 1983.

Sepe, S.J., Marks, J.S., Oakley, G.P., and Manley, A.F. Genetic services in the United States. *Journal of the American Medical Association*, 1982, *248*, 1733-1735.

Shepard, D.S. and Thompson, M.S. First principles of cost-effectiveness analysis in health. *Public Health Reports*, 1979, *94*, 535-543.

Simpson, J.L., Golbus, M.S., Martin, A.O., and Sarto, G.E. *Genetics in obstetrics and gynecology*. New York: Grune & Stratton, 1982.

Sommers, K.B. *Cost-effectiveness analysis for policymaking in prevention: Issues and questions*. Background paper for Institute of Medicine, April, 1984.

Stokey, E. and Zeckhauser, R. *A primer for policy analysis*. New York: W.W. Norton, 1978.

Veatch, R.M. *A theory of medical ethics*. New York: Basic Books, Inc., 1981.

Veatch, R.M. Is autonomy an outmoded value? *The Hastings Center Report*, 1984, *14*, 38-40.

Weinstein, M.C., Fineberg, H.V., Elstein, A.S., Frazier, H.S., Neuhauser, D., Neutra, R.R., and McNeil, B.J. *Clinical decision analysis*. Philadelphia: W.B. Saunders, 1980.

Wortman, P.M. and Saxe, L. Assessment of medical technology: Methodological considerations. Appendix C. *Strategies for medical technology assessment*. Congress of the United
States. Washington, D. C.: Office of Technology Assessment, 1982, 127-149.
Ziporyn, T. Medical decision making: Analyzing options in the face of uncertainty. *Journal
of the American Medical Association*, 1983, *249*, 2133-2142.

Appendix 1

Glossary and Abbreviations

Acetylcholinesterase (AChE): An enzyme catalyzing the hydrolysis of acetylcholine.
AChE is present in increased amounts in the amniotic fluid of fetuses affected with
neural tube defects.

Alpha-fetoprotein (AFP): A protein produced by the fetus and found in the amniotic
fluid. The amounts of alpha-fetoprotein increase during normal pregnancy up to the
34th week, but abnormally high levels are found under certain benign (i.e., multiple
births) or serious conditions (i.e., neural tube defects, fetal death). The protein is
also found in the mother's blood. AF-AFP: alpha-fetoprotein in the amniotic fluid;
MSAFP: alpha-fetoprotein in the maternal serum.

Amniocentesis: A procedure, generally performed during the second trimester of
pregnancy, whereby amniotic fluid is withdrawn from the amniotic sac surrounding
the fetus. Analysis of amniotic fluid may provide important diagnostic information
about fetal anomalies.

Cost-Effectiveness Analysis (CEA): Cost-effectiveness analysis is a means of determining the most efficient allocation of limited resources, by assignment of the ratio
of benefits to resources consumed for each alternative choice followed by selection
of alternatives in ascending order of cost:benefit ratio until resources are exhausted
(Ziporyn, 1983).

Decision Analysis (DA): Decision analysis is a systematic approach to analyzing
options under conditions of uncertainty for the purpose of making decisions. Decisions and outcomes in a clinical situation can be evaluated more clearly through a
decision tree (see Part II, Section B).

Neural Tube Defect (NTD): Neural tube defects are a group of malformations that
result from the abnormal closure of the neural tube, an early fetal structure, during
development. The deficits resulting from abnormal closure depend on the location
of the defect. Abnormal closure in the head region results in anencephaly, which is
uniformly fatal; abnormal closure in the spinal cord region results in spina bifida
(SB), which is compatible with life but carries a wide range of degrees of impairment
(see description of the disorder in text).

Probability: Probability is the chance that a given event will occur. Any event with
a probability of "1" has absolute certainty, any event with a probability of "0" has
absolute impossibility, and all other events are numbered somewhere between,
according to their likelihood of occurrence. Thus probability is the ratio of a specified
event to total events.

Real time ultrasound: A type of ultrasonography in which images are generated rapidly and repetitively to represent many per second of the same section through tissue, so that motion of interfaces can be observed.

Sensitivity analysis: This is a test in which a single variable is varied across a range to see how the results are affected. For example, in evaluating hepatitis B immunization, one might assume the efficacy of the vaccine to be 87.5%; that is, there is a 1 in 8 chance of getting hepatitis despite the vaccination. Thus, it is a means of testing a variety of possibilities in a clinical situation, by taking different numbers for differing conditions and analyzing the outcomes for each one and eventually determining the most likely result for a particular situation (Ziporyn, 1983).

Technology Assessment (TA): Technology assessment is designed to determine the degree to which a particular technology performs the function for which it is devised and thus to provide the basic information for its appropriate use. Technology assessment will determine the efficacy (measure of benefit under ideal conditions), effectiveness (measure of benefit under average conditions of use), and safety (acceptability of risk in a specified situation) (see Banta et al., 1981).

Utility: This is the economist's term for value. When more than two final outcomes are possible, "utility assessment" allows the decision maker to come up with a numerical scale (a "utility scale") explicitly denoting the strength of the preferences. Because they are based on subjective preference, utilities can vary from person to person.

Appendix 2

Roster of Prenatal Diagnosis Project Subgroup of the Working Groups on Disease Prevention and Health Promotion and Early Life and Adolescent Health Policy

Elena O. Nightingale, M.D., Ph.D.,
Chair
Lecturer, Division of Health Policy
  Research and Education
Harvard University
Boston, MA
and
Special Advisor to the President
Carnegie Corporation of New York
New York, NY
and
Adjunct Professor of Pediatrics
Georgetown University Medical
  Center
Washington, DC

Mary Ellen Avery, M.D.
Professor of Pediatrics
Harvard Medical School
Children's Hospital Medical Center
Boston, MA

Fredric Frigoletto, Jr., M.D.
Professor, Department of Obstetrics
  and Gynecology
Harvard Medical School
and
Chief, Maternal-Fetal Medicine
Brigham & Women's Hospital
Boston, MA

Mary L. Kiely, Ph.D.*
Macy Fellow, Division of Health
  Policy Research and Education
Harvard University
John F. Kennedy School of
  Government
Cambridge, MA

Samuel A. Latt, M.D.
Professor of Pediatrics
Harvard Medical School
Children's Hospital
Boston, MA

Alexander Leaf, M.D.
Ridley Watts Professor of Preventive
  Medicine
and
Professor of Medicine
Harvard Medical School
Massachusetts General Hospital
Boston, MA

Barbara J. McNeil, M.D., Ph.D.
Professor of Radiology and Clinical
  Epidemiology
Harvard Medical School
Brigham & Women's Hospital
Boston, MA

Susan B. Meister, Ph.D., R.N.
Associate in Health Policy
Harvard Medical School
Division of Health Policy Research
  and Education
Boston, MA
and
Director, Health Services Research
Children's Hospital and Health Center
San Diego, CA

Julius B. Richmond, M.D.
Director, Division of Health Policy
  Research and Education
and
John D. MacArthur Professor of
  Health Policy and Management
Harvard University
Boston, MA

Kenneth Ryan, M.D.
Chairman, Department of Obstetrics
  and Gynecology
Brigham & Women's Hospital
Boston, MA

Donald S. Shepard, Ph.D.
Associate Professor, Center for the
  Analysis of Health Practices
Harvard School of Public Health
Boston, MA

Richard Zeckhauser, Ph.D.
Professor of Political Economy
John F. Kennedy School of
  Government
Cambridge, MA

---

*Currently: Program Associate
  Carnegie Corporation of New York

Appendix 3a

Working Group on EARLY LIFE AND ADOLESCENT HEALTH POLICY

Julius B. Richmond, M.D., Chairman
Professor of Health Policy
and Director
Division of Health Policy Research
and Education
Harvard University

Mary Ellen Avery, M.D.
Professor of Pediatrics
Children's Hospital Medical Center
Boston, MA

William Beardslee, M.D.
Clinical Director
Department of Psychiatry
Children's Hospital Medical Center
Judge Baker Guidance Center
Boston, MA

Bettye M. Caldwell
Donaghey Professor of Education
Center for Child Development and
  Education
College of Education
University of Arkansas at Little Rock
Little Rock, AR

Stephen Davidson, Ph.D.
Director, Health Management
  Programs
Boston University School of
  Management
Boston, MA

Leon Eisenberg, M.D.
Chairman, Department of Social
  Medicine and Health Policy
Harvard Medical School
Boston, MA

Fredric D. Frigoletto, M.D.
Professor, Department of Obstetrics
  and Gynecology
Harvard Medical School
Chief, Maternal-Fetal Medicine
Brigham & Women's Hospital
Boston, MA

32

Steven L. Gortmaker, Ph.D.
Associate Professor and Acting
    Chairman
Department of Behavioral Science
Harvard School of Public Health
Boston, MA

*Bernard Guyer, M.D., M.P.H.**
Director, Family Health Services
Mass. Department of Public Health
Boston, MA

Beatrix A. Hamburg, M.D.
Professor of Psychiatry and Pediatrics
Mt. Sinai School of Medicine
Division of Child and Adolescent
    Psychiatry
New York, NY

David Hemenway, Ph.D.
Lecturer in Political Economy
Dept. of Health Policy and
    Management
Harvard School of Public Health
Boston, MA

Constance Horgan, Sc.D.
(Visiting Member)
Christopher Walker Fellow
Center for Health Policy and
    Management
John F. Kennedy School of
    Government
Cambridge, MA

Jerome Kagan, Ph.D.
Professor of Human Developmental
    and Social Relations
Department of Psychology
Harvard University
Cambridge, MA

Lorraine Klerman, Dr. P.H.
Professor of Public Health
Department of Epidemiology and
    Public Health
Yale School of Medicine
New Haven, CT

Milton Kotelchuck, Ph.D.
Assistant Professor of Social
    Medicine and Health Policy
Division of Health Policy Research
    and Education
Boston, MA

George A. Lamb, M.D.
Director, Family Health and
    Community Epidemiology
    Department, Health and Hospitals
Boston City Hospital
Boston, MA

Robert Masland, M.D.
Associate Professor of Pediatrics
Harvard Medical School
Children's Hospital Medical Center
Chief, Division of Adolescent—
    Young Adult Medicine
Boston, MA

Donald Medearis, M.D.
Chief, Children's Services
Massachusetts General Hospital
Boston, MA

Martha Minow, J.D.
Assistant Professor
Harvard Law School
Cambridge, MA

---

*Currently: Associate Professor,
Department of Maternal and Child
Health
Harvard School of Public Health
Boston, MA

Elena O. Nightingale, M.D., Ph.D.
Lecturer, Division of Health Policy
  Research and Education
Harvard University
Boston, MA
and
Special Advisor to the President
Carnegie Corporation of New York
New York, NY
and
Adjunct Professor of Pediatrics
Georgetown University School
  of Medicine
Washington, D.C.

Judith S. Palfrey, M.D.
Co-Director, Division of Ambulatory
  Medicine
Children's Hospital Medical Center
Boston, MA

Philip J. Porter, M.D.
Associate Professor of Pediatrics
Harvard Medical School
Division of Health Policy Research
  and Education
Boston, MA

John W. Rowe, M.D.
Deputy Director, Division of Health
  Policy Research and Education
Director, Gerontology Division
Division on Aging
Beth Israel Hospital
Boston, MA

Kenneth Ryan, M.D.
Chairman, Department of Obstetrics
  and Gynecology
Brigham and Women's Hospital
Boston, MA

Lisbeth Schorr
Lecturer
Harvard Medical School
Boston, MA

Deborah Klein Walker, Ed.D.
Associate Professor
Department of Behavioral Sciences
Harvard School of Public Health
Boston, MA

Paul Wise, M.D.
Harvard Medical School
Division of Health Policy Research
  and Education
Boston, MA

Michael Yogman, M.D.
Director
Infant Health and Development
  Program
Children's Hospital Medical School
Boston, MA

Division Staff

John Butler, Ed.D.
Executive Officer
Working Group on Early Life and
  Adolescent Health Policy
Children's Hospital Medical Center
Boston, MA

Susan B. Meister, Ph.D., R.N.
Associate in Health Policy
Division of Health Policy Research
  and Education
and
Director, Health Services Research
Children's Hospital and Health Center
San Diego, CA

Stephen Buka
Research Assistant
Division of Health Policy Research
  and Education
Boston, MA

Victoria Mitchell
Secretary to Early Life Working
  Group
Division of Health Policy Research
  and Education
Boston, MA

Appendix 3b

Working Group on HEALTH PROMOTION AND DISEASE PREVENTION

Alexander Leaf, M.D., Chairman
Chairman, Department of Preventive
Medicine and Clinical Epidemiology
Harvard Medical School
Massachusetts General Hospital
Boston, MA

Charles A. Czeisler, M.D., Ph.D.
Executive Officer
Assistant Professor of Medicine
Harvard Medical School
Director
Neuroendocrinology Laboratory
Brigham and Women's Hospital
Boston, MA

David Calkins, M.D.
Assistant in Medicine
Beth Israel Hospital
Instructor in Medicine
Harvard Medical School
Division of Health Policy
Research and Education
Harvard University
Boston, MA

Paul D. Cleary, Ph.D.
Assistant Professor of Social
  Medicine and Health Policy
Harvard Medical School
B.I.A.C.
Beth Israel Hospital
Boston, MA

Lois Cohen, Ph.D.
Chief, Office of Planning, Evaluation
  and Communication
National Institute of Dental Research
National Institutes of Health
Bethesda, MD

Philip S. Coonley, Ph.D.
U.S. Department of Transportation
Research and Special Program
  Administration
Transportation System Center
Cambridge, MA

Gregory Curfman, M.D.
Assistant Professor of Preventive
  Medicine and Clinical
  Epidemiology
Harvard Medical School
Massachusetts General Hospital
Boston, MA

G. William Dec, M.D.
Instructor in Medicine
Harvard Medical School
Assistant in Medicine
Massachusetts General Hospital
Boston, MA

Howard Fishbein, Dr.P.H.
Director, Health Promotion Sciences
Center for Health Promotion and
  Environmental Disease Prevention
Massachusetts Dept. of Public Health
Boston, MA

36

Part II
Analytic Methods: Technical Reports

A. Literature on Prenatal Screening for Neural Tube Defects: Standards of Technology Assessment[1]

Mary L. Kiely, Ph.D.
Susan B. Meister, Ph.D., R.N.

Technology assessment is one method for evaluating medical tests and procedures. It begins with identifying what is known about the capabilities of a test or procedure, and goes on to identify the best uses of the technology. The analysis presented here measures the tests and procedures used in prenatal screening for neural tube defects against three standards of technology assessment: efficacy, effectiveness, and safety.

Hamburg (1981) described three applications of the results of technology assessment:

• to insure that technologies with probable benefit and acceptable risk are made available;
• to constrain the use of less acceptable technologies; and
• to guide appropriate use of new and old technologies.

With these goals in mind, we designed an analysis of the literature concerned with the tests and procedures used in prenatal screening for neural tube defects.[2] Wortman and Saxe (1978), in a major review of methods for technology assessment, identified literature review as a method of determining what is known about the efficacy, effectiveness, and safety of medical technologies. We did not expect to establish the absolute efficacy, effectiveness, and safety of these tests and procedures. Rather, we intended to assess the breadth and depth of the literature about them, using these three standards of technology assessment as a benchmark to determine if there is a consensus among investigators on the use of these diagnostic tools.

Our question was *how well have the standards been applied to these tests and procedures*? We expected to find gaps in the literature, and our premise was that identifying these gaps was important to policy analysis—because unrecognized shortfalls in knowledge could lead to unrecognized errors in policies.

It is important to recognize the limitations of using published literature as our data. Delays in publication and rapid developments in the technologies studied will no doubt outdate some of our substantive conclusions in short order. Even so, this

37

analysis illustrates one way of producing substantial knowledge for policy analyses and forms the basis for further analyses, such as by consensus panels of experts in the field.

1. Problem for Analysis

Before we could assess how well the literature addresses the standards of technology assessment, we had to select definitions of those standards. Technology assessment is well established and there are many opinions about what the standards mean. We rely primarily on Banta, Behney and Willems' (1981) definitions, and describe our interpretation of their concepts below.

The Standard of Efficacy. The efficacy of a test or procedure is the theoretical probability of deriving benefit from using a technology. Efficacy is virtually a "best case" issue because the probability of benefit is estimated by assuming that the test is used under optimal circumstances.

Four principal criteria determine efficacy: benefit to be achieved, medical problem, population affected, conditions of use (Banta et al., 1981; Fineberg et al., 1977). The benefits of a diagnostic technology are determined by five criteria:
• Technical Capability—Is the technology reliable and does it provide accurate information?
• Diagnostic Accuracy—Does the technology provide an accurate diagnosis?
• Diagnostic Impact—Does the technology replace other technologies?
• Therapeutic Impact—Do the results obtained from the technology affect the planning and delivery of health care?
• Patient Outcome—Does the technology contribute to the improved health of the patient?[3]

Therefore, our analysis was designed to describe how well the literature for *each* test and procedure used in prenatal screening for neural tube defects addresses the five criteria. It is equally important to do the same analysis for the tests and procedures as a *group*.

Banta et al. (1981) observed that the efficacy of a specific technology can be determined only in relation to the medical condition for which it is applied. In this analysis, we consider the tests and techniques only as they are used in prenatal screening for neural tube defects, although several are used in the evaluation of a variety of other medical problems.

Even with the optimal conditions assumed under efficacy, the performance of a test or procedure can vary according to which group or population is tested. For example, a test for Disease X would produce a higher diagnostic yield in a population with a higher incidence of Disease X. Therefore, efficacy is not independent of the population being tested (Banta et al., 1981).

In this analysis, the population being tested changes with each test. Only women with test results suggesting increased probability of a neural tube defect in the fetus will be offered the next test in the screening program.

We designed the analysis to track how well the literature describes efficacy for several groups of women; those at increased risk and continuing screening, those at increased risk and declining further screening, and those at decreased risk and eliminated from screening. Medical problem and population affected are often synonymous. We usually discuss them together, under a single heading.

The criterion of conditions of use relates the outcomes of using a technology to the situation in which it is used because all medical technologies are designed to be

38

used in a particular way. Banta et al. (1981) observed that outcomes are affected by the abilities of the people who use the technology, the setting in which they use it, and the quality of the materials that are used.

Each test and procedure analyzed here requires certain skills, clinical situations, equipment, and laboratory materials. We were particularly interested in this issue because it can dramatically alter policy options. For example, if a test only obtains high efficacy when used by people with ten years of experience, then it will only be effective for use in the general population if such people exist in appropriate numbers.

The Standard of Effectiveness. The effectiveness of a technology is the measure of its benefit under average or general conditions of use. This measure differs from efficacy, which is determined by the probability of benefit under ideal conditions of use.

The history of prenatal screening for neural tube defects illustrates a stepwise relationship between efficacy and effectiveness. In the early 1970s, Brock and his colleagues developed the initial screening test for maternal serum alpha-fetoprotein, based on their observation that alpha-fetoprotein concentrations are greatly elevated in maternal blood when a fetus has an open neural tube defect (Brock and Sutcliffe, 1972). The efficacy of the MSAFP test was studied in university hospitals, using carefully controlled situations. Once efficacy had been demonstrated, the effectiveness of the test was examined in a large-scale screening program that incorporated 19 clinical centers in the United Kingdom.

In our literature review, we found that many reports discuss (or are pertinent to) both efficacy and effectiveness. We report our results in this fashion as well, speaking first about the theoretical efficacy of each technology and then the practical effectiveness of it.

The Standard of Safety. Banta et al. (1981) describe the safety of medical technologies as "causing no undue harm," and point out that estimating safety requires making a judgment about the acceptability of risk. Risk can be defined as the probability of having an adverse or untoward outcome. This judgment is made relative to the population under consideration, the medical problem for which the technology is applied, and the conditions of use.

The judgment may be affected by factors that are only indirectly related to the technology, particularly if the technology is part of a series of tests. In prenatal screening for neural tube defects, the primary function of the first test is correct classification of the population into groups that should (and should not) have the next test. The risk at this point is not misdiagnosis but misclassification, because the group classified as not needing another test will be removed from the testing program. Therefore, we designed our analysis to track discussions of both kinds of risk: risk of misclassification, and risk of misdiagnosis.

2. Methodology

Our analysis is limited to information from literature related to prenatal screening for neural tube defects and published by 1984. We examined reports of basic research, clinical applications, pilot population applications, and analyses of policy issues such as cost-effectiveness. We reviewed original reports and review articles, and assumed statistical accuracy.

We examined the literature to identify how well it addressed the standards of efficacy, effectiveness, and safety. Figure 1 illustrates how we structured our analysis of concordance. Our primary aim was to highlight issues that were not addressed and therefore, our presentation focuses on gaps in the literature rather than on points of concordance.

Figure 1
Structure of the Review

Which of the following issues have not been addressed regarding MSAFP testing, ultrasonographic examination of women with elevated MSAFP, amniocentesis, and AFP/AChE tests on amniotic fluid?

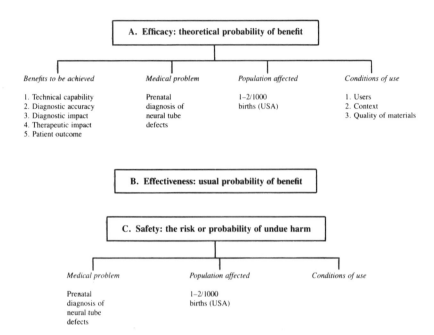

3. Results

Maternal serum alpha-fetoprotein (MSAFP)

Maternal serum alpha-fetoprotein (MSAFP) results from leakage of fetal alpha-fetoprotein (AFP) into maternal blood. In the second trimester of pregnancy, fetal AFP levels are at least 100 times as great as maternal levels (ACOG, 1982). AFP levels are usually greatly elevated when the fetus is affected with an open neural tube defect (NTD) and this elevation should be reflected in maternal serum levels. A blood test for MSAFP, performed between 16 and 18 weeks of gestation, serves as the first test in prenatal screening for neural tube defects.

Efficacy and effectiveness. Technical capability is the first criterion that determines the benefits to be achieved. MSAFP is the initial screening tool and its chief benefit should be an accurate classification of pregnant women according to relative risk of NTDs in the fetus. If a woman has a normal MSAFP level, she will have no further NTD-screening tests. If the MSAFP result is abnormal, the woman will be offered a repeat MSAFP test. A false negative MSAFP (normal MSAFP when the fetus is affected with an NTD) will eliminate a woman from further testing; a false positive MSAFP (abnormal MSAFP when the fetus is not affected with an NTD) will expose a woman to unnecessary further testing.

MSAFP results may be calibrated as either multiples of the normal MSAFP median (MoMdn) or percentiles. Neither method resolves a fundamental problem with this test: MSAFP results are not categorical, they are continuous. There are no discrete cutoff points, rather, those points are established using several methods. This scalar property makes it difficult to interpret borderline values. For example, it is difficult to distinguish between "high normal" values and "low elevated" values. We did not find a consensus in the literature regarding the most useful mode of calibration for this test.

The sensitivity and specificity of MSAFP are different for the two primary forms of NTDs: anencephaly and spina bifida. Goldberg and Oakley (1979) calculated that MSAFP will be elevated for 84% of pregnancies with anencephalic fetuses and 59% of pregnancies with spina bifida fetuses. In other words, the test will give false negative results for 16% of anencephaly and 41% of spina bifida. The test will yield false positive results for 1% of unaffected fetuses. These numbers describe the test performance if the 99th percentile is used to distinguish between normal and elevated MSAFP. A lower cutoff, such as the 95th percentile, will result in identifying more affected fetuses while increasing the number of false positives.

Cutoff points for MoMdn calibrations have also been tested as compromises between maximizing detection rates and minimizing false positive rates. Brock (1981) compared the effects of using 2.0 and 3.0 MoMdn in screening one million hypothetical pregnant women. Assuming that all women follow the screening protocol and that the incidence of NTDs is 1 in 1,000 births, the 2.0 MoMdn cutoff would detect 88% of neural tube defects. This process would require 20,000 amniocentesis procedures, and there would be 300 fetal losses. Under the same assumptions, the 3.0 MoMdn cutoff would detect 68% of neural tube defects, require only 5,000 amniocenteses, and result in 75 fetal losses.

Therefore, the literature suggests that while exact rates may vary between calibration methods, the proportions of false positives and false negatives, the requirements for further testing, and proportions of fetal loss will each shift when the cutoff for the first test is changed.

Others have estimated the relative risk of NTDs associated with specific MSAFP values. Crandall et al. (1978) calculated that if NTD prevalence is 2 per 1,000 births, then an MSAFP value greater than 2.5 MoMdn suggests about 1 chance in 20 that the fetus is affected. Holtzman et al. (1981) found that about 2.7% of women with MSAFP exceeding the 95th percentile will have an affected fetus. Brock's (1981) analysis worked in the opposite direction and found that 90% of the affected pregnancies had MSAFP values greater than or equal to the 98th percentile. Adams et al. (1984) propose that the problem lies in determining the size of two groups (NTD-affected pregnancies and unaffected pregnancies) for *each* MSAFP value. Their mathematical models take small increments in MSAFP and estimate the associated risk of an NTD.

The accuracy of test results also depends on laboratory procedures (ACOG, 1982). Each laboratory must establish its own norms by computing the mean (or median), the first five standard deviations above the mean, and the coefficient of variance on 100 samples for each week of gestation (Crandall et al. 1978). These samples are drawn from pregnant women. The MSAFP values from the women who have normal infants are used to calibrate the test. For our analysis, these stringent laboratory requirements suggest that policy analysis cannot simply apply the sensitivity and specificity of MSAFP. The test can only perform well in large scale applications if there are enough appropriate laboratories to run test results.

Calibration by gestational age is important because the volume of AFP increases during the second trimester of pregnancy. Thus, an MSAFP value that would be considered elevated at 16 weeks gestation would be considered normal later in pregnancy. On the other hand, MSAFP testing should not be done too early in pregnancy. Ferguson-Smith (1979) reported that even fetuses with severe, open forms of NTDs may produce normal MSAFP values before 15 weeks gestation. Therefore, in addition to laboratory requirements, an accurate estimate of gestational age is a prerequisite to obtaining the best test performance.

In terms of the criteria of diagnostic accuracy and impact, MSAFP is not diagnostic of NTDs; it provides only an initial screening. MSAFP values may be elevated in pregnancies with normal twins, fetal death, NTDs or several other congenital disorders.

We identified the primary benefit of MSAFP as accurate classification according to risk of an NTD. Under usual conditions, however, some women with elevated MSAFP results will decline further screening. In this case, the MSAFP result could have diagnostic impact because it is the only test. We found little discussion of this effect of MSAFP in the literature.

MSAFP itself does not have direct therapeutic impact, but abnormal MSAFP alters obstetrical care by establishing an indication for further testing. Whether this outcome is of value depends on factors such as test accuracy, the availability of services, and maternal preferences.

In 1980, the U.S. Food and Drug Administration (FDA) estimated that MSAFP values would affect a hypothetical group of 1,000 women in this manner: 50 will have elevated MSAFP; 30 of those elevations will be maintained in repeat MSAFP tests. Half (15) of those women will have an ultrasonographic examination that fails to explain the elevated MSAFP. One or two of those 15 women will have elevated AFP values in amniotic fluid. One in every 10 women with elevated AFP will have a normal fetus, and 9 will have NTD-affected fetuses (Department of Health and Human Services, 1980).[4] We observed that reports of screening programs focus primarily on women who have all of the tests, offering little insight into outcomes for all other women.

Gardner, Burton, and Johnson (1981) and Sowers and Burton (1982) suggest that low or undetectable MSAFP values may also have clinical significance, and therefore, therapeutic impact. Sowers and Burton found that among 6,360 pregnant women in North Carolina, 159 (2.5%) had MSAFP values below 0.3 MoMdn. Nearly 60% of the women with low values had pregnancies that were less advanced than had been estimated; 4.4% of the women were not pregnant, 12.6% had had fetal loss, and 23.3% had apparently normal pregnancies with accurate estimates of gestational age. Levels below 0.4 MoMdn indicated an increased risk for chromosomal disorders, particularly trisomies such as Down Syndrome. Sowers and Burton (1982) concluded that *low* MSAFP should be considered an indication for repeat testing. We found only two reports of large scale screening programs that described the outcomes for women with low MSAFP.

42

The final determinant of benefit to be achieved is patient outcome. If MSAFP values are accurate, if further screening is available, and if the patient would prefer to have prenatal knowledge of her relative risk of an NTD-affected fetus, MSAFP testing can contribute to her well-being. It is difficult to establish whether or not this statement applies to the fetus as well.

If we consider MSAFP testing alone, without regard to the availability and desirability of further testing, Brock (1982) observes that we should consider the effects of anxiety. He reported that anxiety is likely to follow an elevated test result, and suggested that services such as counseling, education, and support may be necessary. However, if even the suggestion that a pregnancy be screened for a congenital defect causes anxiety, then MSAFP testing affects the psychological outcomes for all women, not just women who eventually have elevated MSAFP values. We found no discussion of the physiological effect of such psychological outcomes.

In considering the medical problem of fetal NTDs, MSAFP is the first test in prenatal diagnosis, but its use depends on the population being tested. For example, the testing may be offered to all women with a family history of NTDs, because they are known to be at higher risk. Alternatively, the testing may be offered to normal-risk women (those with no family history of NTDs). Since about 95% of NTDs occur among normal-risk women, mass screening efforts are usually aimed at the entire pregnant population.

Although the national incidence of NTDs is about 1–2 per 1,000 live births (Goldberg and Oakley, 1979), incidence varies substantially in relation to maternal race, geographic location, and history of NTDs. For example, Greenberg, James and Oakley (1983) found that NTD incidence was 1 per 10,000 among Black women living in the Rocky Mountains and 8 per 10,000 among White women living in Southern Appalachia. For this analysis, Greenberg's findings point out that the incidence of the medical problem may change dramatically with the population receiving NTD screening.

Regardless of the population, the literature includes specific analyses of the optimal conditions of use. Reports describe methods of calibration and reagent preparation, but we found no consensus on calibration issues. Adams et al. (1984) identify a number of factors that affect the interpretation of MSAFP values; gestational age, maternal weight, maternal diabetes, race, and geographic residence. While the authors' mathematical models would improve the interpretation of MSAFP, Adams et al. also point out that the models include data, such as gestational day, which may not be available even in optimal situations.

None of the reports of screening programs describe randomization or control groups (Macri, Haddow, and Weiss, 1979; Macri, Weiss, and Libster, 1979; Gardner, Burton, and Johnson, 1981). We did not find either a report of a randomized clinical trial of the whole screening protocol, or a discussion of why such a trial would be precluded.

Safety. Although the MSAFP testing procedure has the same degree of physiological risk as does any venipuncture performed on a pregnant woman, three other kinds of risk should be considered. First, there is the risk of misclassification. Even under optimal conditions, the accuracy of MSAFP results is affected by NTD incidence, test calibration, knowledge of variables such as gestational age, and the methods used to interpret the results. Although the test will be repeated if initial results are elevated, only Adams et al. (1984) and Goldberg and Oakley (1979)

43

analyzed the manner in which a repeat MSAFP affects the relative risk of misclassification.

Second, although prompt follow-up testing of MSAFP can correct misclassification, pilot screening programs demonstrated that some women will refuse these tests. We found little information about the outcomes of those pregnancies. Finally, although Milunsky and Alpert (1984) point out that women with elevated MSAFP are likely to experience considerable anxiety, the literature also lacks analysis of the supportive services that may be required after MSAFP testing.

Diagnostic ultrasonography

Diagnostic ultrasonography has many applications in obstetrical practice, including evaluation of women with elevated MSAFP. Ultrasonography is used following elevated MSAFP to obtain an accurate assessment of gestational age and to check for the presence of several conditions that may produce elevated MSAFP.

In 1984, the U.S. Department of Health and Human Services published the report of a consensus development conference on diagnostic ultrasonographic imaging in pregnancy. The charge to the consensus group was considerably broader than our questions about the use of ultrasonography as part of prenatal screening for neural tube defects. The consensus group established the types, purposes, and extent of use of ultrasonographic scanning in obstetrics, evaluated the evidence that ultrasonography improves the management and outcomes of pregnancy, described the theoretical and documented risks to mother and fetus, and defined the appropriate indications for use of ultrasonography in obstetrics (Department of Health and Human Services, 1984). The findings of the consensus panel are a primary reference in this section.

Efficacy and effectiveness. Technical capability and diagnostic accuracy are major determinants of the benefit to be achieved through ultrasonography. The technical contribution of this technique to prenatal NTD screening is threefold: to provide an accurate estimate of gestational age, to look for evidence of conditions that can cause elevated MSAFP (i.e., NTDs, multiple gestation, fetal death, other congenital disorders), and, if possible, to estimate the size and location of spina bifida and allow an estimate of the probable severity of the lesion.

Despite dramatic improvements in ultrasonography, diagnostic accuracy varies with gestational age and conditions of use. For example, one form of NTDs (anencephaly) may be detected by ultrasonography as early as the 12th week of gestation, while another form (spina bifida) is not usually visible until the 20th week (ACOG, 1982). This may change, as the resolution of equipment and experience of operators increase.

While there is an upper limit on how finely the ultrasonographic equipment can visualize fetal structures, the skill of the ultrasonographer is another crucial determinant of diagnostic accuracy. The joint effects of equipment and sonographer skill were observed by Roberts et al. (1983). The researchers observed a sharp improvement in diagnosis of spina bifida (from 33.3% to 80%) and marked decrease in false positive rates (from 3.94% to 0.34%) between the first and second year of experience with obstetrical ultrasonography in a university hospital. In fact, the diagnostic ultrasound consensus panel recommended that standards for both equipment and operators should be established.

The accuracy of ultrasonographic estimates of gestational age can also vary. Obstetricians usually depend on maternal history and physical examinations to estimate gestational age; ultrasonography uses precise measurements of fetal structures such as biparietal diameter. While this estimate seems to be especially reliable during the weeks when NTD screening is conducted, even then it may be off by as much as 10 days (ACOG, 1981). This potential for error merits attention because a sizable proportion of women having prenatal NTD screening will have gestational age adjusted by ultrasonography. For example, Bennett et al. (1982) reported that gestational age was recalibrated for 25% of women having ultrasonography after two elevated MSAFP tests. The probability of error at this step in screening is important because testing stops if the MSAFP values are normal for the revised gestational age. Watson et al. (1983) observed that this application of ultrasonographic findings calls for more clinical research.

Diagnostic impact is another criterion for determining benefit to be achieved. Ultrasonography is not always considered to be diagnostic in prenatal screening for NTDs. The function of the procedure is similar to that of MSAFP testing; both tests serve to classify women according to relative risk of an NTD and establish indications for further testing. ACOG (1982) estimated that 30-40% of women with two elevated MSAFP results will have "negative" ultrasonographic findings, that is, singleton fetuses of expected gestational age and no apparent condition to explain the elevated MSAFP values. These women would be offered amniocentesis to measure AFP and AChE.

The results of ultrasonography are not completely accurate. The NIH Consensus group pointed out that it is still difficult to visualize NTD lesions. For example, while ultrasonography will correct some of the false positives from MSAFP, one form of NTD (spina bifida) is difficult to visualize and 5-10% of such lesions may be missed (Harris and Read, 1981; Hobbins et al., 1982). Thus, some women with affected fetuses will have negative ultrasonographic findings—but these women would be referred for amniocentesis.

Ultrasonography would have diagnostic impact if it replaced amniocentesis and served as a final test when an NTD is visualized. We did not find reports of clinical trials, but Brock (1983) described the patterns of referral to amniocentesis following visualization of an NTD. Over the four years of the study the rate of referral for amniocentesis declined; nonetheless, the majority of patients (55% of suspected anencephaly and 76% of suspected spina bifida cases) were referred. These results suggest that while confidence in ultrasonographic imaging increased, clinicians still preferred to have ultrasonographic findings confirmed with amniocentesis for AFP measurement.

Hobbins et al. (1982) proposed another route to increasing the diagnostic impact of ultrasonography. They suggest adding a more sophisticated version of the procedure for women who have elevated AFP after amniocentesis. The additional ultrasonography would be used to correct false positives from AFP and to obtain more information about the size and level of NTD lesions. We found no reports of clinical trials to establish the efficacy or effectiveness of this screening protocol.

Therapeutic impact also determines the benefit to be gained from ultrasonography. The procedure would affect obstetrical care by establishing either a reason for elevated MSAFP or an indication for further testing. In both cases, obstetrical care would be altered. The consensus group pointed out that ultrasonographic information is useful when it decreases the clinician's uncertainty about a diagnosis (DHHS, 1984).

Finally, ultrasonography in prenatal screening for NTDs would improve patient outcomes if the results were accurate and women had access to indicated services. The consensus group concluded that ultrasonography improves obstetrical care when it is used for an accepted medical indication, although randomized clinical trials will be necessary to determine the efficacy of routine ultrasonographic scanning during pregnancy (DHHS, 1984).

It is possible that ultrasonography could affect outcomes in other ways. For example, Fletcher and Evans (1983) observed two ultrasonographic procedures and concluded that the examination itself can affect parents' views of the value and acceptability of the fetus. Reading and Cox (1982) studied a small sample of young, white, low-risk maternity patients. The pilot study suggested an interaction between what kind of information is provided for the patient and the patient's reports of feeling worried or uncertain. The consensus group found the literature on psychological effects of ultrasonography to be limited and suggested further study in this area (DHHS, 1984). The group pointed out that we need to know more than whether or not such effects occur, but also if they are positive or negative.

During prenatal screening for NTDs, ultrasonography will be offered to women with two elevated MSAFP results. These women are thought to be at greater risk for NTDs, although not all of them will have affected fetuses. The size of the population and the relative risk of NTDs will vary according to the family histories of the women and the cutoffs used in calibrating the MSAFP tests.

The conditions for using ultrasonographic scanning involve at least the ultrasonographic equipment and the operator. The consensus group noted the rapid development and distribution of the equipment and the lack of uniform requirements for training and education of operators, and concluded that it is very difficult to establish the actual conditions of use for ultrasonography (DHHS, 1984). The group went on to recommend ways to improve the situation, but for now, the literature can only describe what kinds of equipment should be used and what kinds of training ought to be required for operators, whether ultrasonographers or physicians.

Safety. The safety of ultrasonographic imaging during pregnancy has been thoroughly examined by the NIH Consensus group. The group recognized that many of the studies of the risk posed by ultrasonography have methodological flaws, and that it can be difficult to interpret the meaning of biological effects demonstrated *in vitro*. The group also observed that the effects of exposure of the fetus to ultrasonography *in utero* may be subtle and delayed until long after birth, making it difficult to relate them to the procedure.

Based on the literature on structural and biological alterations, and dose-effect relationships, the consensus group concluded that the absence of evidence of risk is not sufficient to establish what intensities or durations of ultrasonographic exposure are safe. The group emphasized the importance of improving dosimetry for ultrasonography and conducting both biological and long-term developmental studies of the effects of the procedure.

Amniocentesis for measurement of alpha-fetoprotein (AFP) and the acetylcholinesterase (AChE) assay

Patients are referred for amniocentesis to detect a variety of congenital and genetic defects. The procedure is essentially the same regardless of the problem under consideration, although the timing of the procedure with respect to the gestational age of the fetus may vary. Amniocentesis is used in prenatal screening for NTDs because amniotic fluid permits a more accurate estimate of AFP levels than does maternal serum.

Amniocentesis is performed after two elevated MSAFP results and examination of fetal structures by ultrasonography. The procedure involves the insertion of a 3½ inch needle through the abdominal wall to withdraw fluid from the amniotic sac surrounding the fetus. For the prenatal detection of neural tube defects, the procedure is usually performed between the 16th and 20th week of gestation (NICHHD, 1979).

In this context, amniocentesis permits two final screening tests. These tests, amniotic fluid alpha-fetoprotein (AF-AFP) and acetylcholinesterase (AChE) are discussed in the following sections. The discussion sometimes returns to amniocentesis, when aspects of the procedure itself are relevant.

Efficacy and effectiveness. The technical capability and diagnostic accuracy of AF-AFP and AChE affect the benefits to be achieved. Greatly elevated amniotic fluid AFP levels are considered to be more accurate in diagnosing NTDs than are MSAFP elevations since AF-AFP measures concentration of the protein directly in the amniotic fluid. Accuracy is subject to some of the same testing problems associated with the measurement of MSAFP. Both the mean and the median have been used to define calibration scales.

Reports on the diagnostic accuracy of the test vary: elevated AF-AFP has been used to identify 80% of anencephaly and 70% of spina bifida (Crandall et al., 1978); while other reports suggest that elevated AF-AFP is a highly reliable indicator of fetal pathology, some of which are neural tube defects (Leonard, 1981). In one hypothetical analysis of 100,000 women, false positive rates for the AF-AFP test were estimated to be 0.034%, or 6 out of 1,751 tests performed on singleton pregnancies (Layde et al., 1979). Brock (1981) reported sensitivities for the test of 97.6% for open spina bifida and 98.2% of anencephaly, with a false positive rate of 0.79%. In each study, the majority of the false positives were associated with other severe congenital defects, such as exomphalos or congenital nephrosis, as well as fetal death. False positive rates increase significantly when measurements are made on samples grossly contaminated with blood (Smith, 1982).

As with MSAFP, inaccurate estimates of gestational age are associated with increased false negative rates. Layde's study (1979) estimated false negative rates of 9.8% or 6 of 61 affected fetuses. False negatives also include closed neural tube defects, which do not release AFP into the surrounding amniotic fluid (ACOG, 1982).

The primary benefit of the acetylcholinesterase (AChE) assay is to provide further evidence for or against the presence of a neural tube defect. Since parents will be faced with the decision of either terminating or continuing the pregnancy, accuracy of this test is of particular importance. Measurement of AChE can complement the AF-AFP test to increase accuracy.

The acetylcholinesterases are enzymes that break down the neurotransmitter acetylcholine, and are located primarily in the cells of the brain and central nervous system. Their role in prenatal NTD screening was described in the Report of the Collaborative Acetylcholinesterase Study (1981). Developing and exposed nerve terminals release AChE into the extracellular space from which it then passes into the cerebrospinal fluid. Some AChE also filters into the fetal plasma, but is absent from adult circulation. Thus, amniotic fluid AChE may be considered a "feto-specific" protein, derived primarily from exposed nerve terminals and cerebrospinal fluid. A specific AChE is found in association with open neural tube defects, including anencephaly and open spina bifida.

47

The identification of AChE is complicated by the presence of high levels of non-specific cholinesterases. Two methods have been developed to distinguish AChE from the nonspecific cholinesterases: a quantitative method and a qualitative method.

Although the quantitative method is rapid and can be automated, a number of studies have reported a high rate of false positive AChE results when certain reagents are used in the presence of samples contaminated with blood (Smith, 1982). A direct assay of AChE activity with different reagents and a nonspecific cholinesterase inhibitor gives fewer false positive results, but problems still exist with samples that are severely contaminated with blood (Dale et al., 1981).

The qualitative method relies on the separation of AChE and nonspecific cholin-esterase by polyacrylamide gel electrophoresis. The individual bands of protein are visualized by precipitation and staining (Haddow et al., 1981; Beuamah et al., 1980; Read et al., 1982). Positive identification of individual bands as either AChE or non-specific cholinesterase is confirmed by simultaneous electrophoresis of samples previously incubated with specific inhibitors of each enzyme.

Smith (1982) estimates the test to be more than 99% sensitive for anencephaly and open spina bifida. Most false positive results are associated with samples grossly contaminated with blood (Seller and Cole, 1980; Wald and Cuckle, 1981), although a few false positives have been attributed to contamination with uterine wall tissue (Smith, 1982). In general, however, the AChE test is much less sensitive to blood contamination than is the AF-AFP assay. False negatives are infrequent; only 4 of 813 NTD pregnancies in one major study. Other fetal conditions, including exom-phalos, intrauterine death, and Turner's Syndrome, are associated with elevated AChE activity, but samples from pregnancies with closed spina bifida are not (Dale et al., 1981).

In terms of diagnostic impact, amniocentesis itself is not a diagnostic procedure, but simply a means for collecting amniotic fluid for the analysis of the component cells and macromolecules. Amniocentesis affects diagnostic accuracy indirectly, because accurate measurements of AF-AFP and AChE depend to a large extent on the quality of the sample obtained (e.g., bloody vs. clear fluid).

For those fetuses that do not present evidence of some form of NTD on ultrason-ography, amniotic fluid AFP measurement is considered the most effective diagnostic test in the series. Results of the AChE assay also have significant diagnostic impact. The test was developed to provide secondary confirmation of a positive AF-AFP test result, and to clarify those AFP results where validity is in question because of the condition of the sample obtained through amniocentesis. Therefore, the results of AF-AFP and AChE present the clinician and pregnant woman with the best available estimate of the risk of an NTD.

In a U.K. Collaborative Study, the presence of a specific AChE in conjunction with a positive test for elevated AFP indicated a 16-fold increase in the risk of having a fetus with an open NTD (Wald and Cuckle, 1981). The actual risk was found to depend on birth incidence and the reason a woman is sent for amniocentesis. By using a birth incidence for NTDs of 2 per 1,000, the risks for open spina bifida when both AF-AFP and AChE results are positive are estimated to be 288:1 for those women referred because of a single elevated MSAFP (2.5 times the normal median between 16-18 weeks gestation), 80:1 for women referred because of a previous birth of an NTD infant, and 8:1 for women referred for other reasons (Wald and Cuckle, 1981). The odds are estimated to be much lower if the samples are contaminated with fetal blood (36:1, 10:1, and 1:1, respectively); and much higher if contaminated

48

with maternal blood (958:1, 265:1, and 26:1, respectively). The AChE band also is present in some cases of intrauterine death, exomphalos, extrophy of cloaca, Turner's syndrome, fetus papyraceous, prune belly syndrome, omphalocele/gastroschisis, and frontal encephalocele (Brock and Hayward, 1980; Wald and Cuckle, 1981).

The absence of AChE in a sample contaminated with blood and showing elevated levels of AFP, on the other hand, places the validity of the AFP test in question. For example, in a study of 200 pregnancies, Milunsky and Sapirstein (1982) were able to reclassify correctly 89% of normal pregnancies with elevated AF-AFP by demonstrating the absence of AChE on polyacrylamide gels. Thus, this test has considerable importance in reassuring women who might otherwise have faced termination of pregnancy.

Therapeutic impact and effects on patient outcomes are the final criteria for determining benefit to be achieved. Amniocentesis affects obstetrical care both directly and indirectly. Directly, complications of the procedure, such as fetal injury, maternal injury or puncture of the placenta, may require therapeutic intervention or alter plans for delivery. Indirectly, a normal AFP value would indicate an unaffected fetus, a contraindication to any therapeutic intervention, whereas an elevated AFP and presence or absence of AChE band permit the risks of an NTD-affected infant to be calculated more precisely. All parents should be offered counseling and those with a high risk for an affected infant are generally given the option of terminating the pregnancy. Parents not desiring termination of the pregnancy should be counseled about how and when to prepare for the birth of an affected child. Perhaps the greatest potential of the complementary AChE assay in the prenatal diagnosis of NTDs is in those cases where AF-AFP is positive, but the quality of the sample obtained through amniocentesis is in question.

The population and medical problem affected would be women who have had two elevated MSAFP results and ultrasonography that did not explain those elevations. They are presumed to have a high risk of NTDs, although the degree of risk is a function of family history and the technical performance of the preceding tests.

The literature addresses conditions of use in relation to amniocentesis, AF-AFP and AChE. According to Benacerraf and Frigoletto (1983), in most medical centers amniocentesis is performed with the aid of an ultrasonographer and an obstetrician. The ultrasonographer locates the fetus and chooses the appropriate site for needle insertion. The needle is then placed blindly through the abdominal wall, assuming the fetus has not moved within the amniotic cavity before or during insertion. Several studies have shown a lower incidence of multiple punctures and bloody taps when ultrasonography is performed just before amniocentesis (Lele, Carmody, Hurd, and O'Leary, 1982; Mennuti, Brummond, Crombleholm, Schwarz, and Arvan, 1980), while others have found no difference (Verp and Gerbie, 1981; Golbus et al., 1979).

Benacerraf and Frigoletto (1983) showed in a series of 232 consecutive taps that real-time ultrasonography used *throughout* the procedure to keep the needle in view resulted in clear fluid being obtained with a single insertion more often than was previously recorded in the literature, and gave the lowest reported incidence of bloody taps, dry taps, and multiple insertions during amniocentesis.

As with MSAFP, the literature gives some specific information on the optimal conditions for AF-AFP determinations. As with many tests, the purity of the reagents used and the experience of the technical personnel performing the test are of great importance. The state of the sample, i.e., whether clear fluid or contaminated with blood, also affects the sensitivity of the test (Smith, 1982). Calibration issues are still under debate. Constructing a "normal" value range is one of the most important issues for each laboratory performing this test.

Optimal conditions for AChE assays have also been described. The AChE test requires the use of a synthetic substrate and an inhibitor for nonspecific cholinesterases. For the quantitative method, the direct assay for AChE activity uses acetylthiocholine as substrate. Lysivane (ethopropazine hydrochloride) is used as the nonspecific cholinesterase inhibitor since it has been shown to give fewer false positives than the inhibitor BW2S4C51 (Smith, 1982).

The qualitative method relies more on the quality and sensitivity of the polyacrylamide gels. Thinner gels have been found to give better resolution. Gel banding patterns on normal pregnancy amniotic fluid should always be included as internal controls, as well as the positive identification of individual bands by use of specific enzyme inhibitors (Smith, 1982).

Again, the quality of the reagents used and the experience of the laboratory and its personnel are important factors in the outcome and reliability of the AChE test results.

Safety. The issue of safety focuses primarily on the risk of fetal injury during amniocentesis and the risk of spontaneous abortion following the procedure. These factors, in turn, have been shown to be related to the gestational age of the fetus, the gauge of the needle, the number of needle insertions, the number of times a woman undergoes the procedure, and whether ultrasonography is used before or during the procedure, or is not used at all.

The most significant problem associated with amniocentesis is the risk of spontaneous miscarriage after the procedure (NICHHD, 1979). In a study conducted by the National Institute for Child Health and Human Development (NICHHD, 1976), fetal loss among women having three or more amniocentesis procedures was twice as great as among those having only two procedures. Reducing the incidence of multiple insertions and bloody taps has been shown by Epley et al. (1979), and Varma (1981) to lower the rate of post-amniocentesis complications, including injury and miscarriage. In 1979, fetal injury due to amniocentesis was estimated to be as high as 9 percent (Epley et al. 1979). However, in a comparative study of 1,040 midtrimester amniocentesis subjects and 992 controls, who did not undergo amniocentesis, there was no statistical difference in rates of fetal loss for the groups (NICHHD, 1976). This study used information from nine clinical centers performing amniocentesis, and thus addressed the technical capability under conditions of use which were average for medical centers.

Fetomaternal bleeding, or the leakage of fetal blood into the maternal circulation, can be associated with amniocentesis. Lele et al. (1982) found a fetal death rate of 16.6% among patients experiencing fetomaternal bleeding after amniocentesis, compared with 1.1% among patients without evidence of fetomaternal bleeding. Fetal injury may also occur, usually as a result of puncturing the fetus with the needle during the procedure. Such injuries may be prevented by simultaneous monitoring of fetal location by ultrasonography.

Controlled clinical studies addressing the efficacy of amniocentesis have shown that safety can be optimized by following certain procedures. For example:

• Benacerraf and Frigoletto (1983) have shown that monitoring with real-time ultrasonography to keep the needle in view throughout amniocentesis significantly reduces both the risk of fetal injury during the procedure, and of spontaneous abortion afterwards. This procedure not only decreases the number of needle insertions required for a successful tap, but effectively limits the number of times a woman must undergo amniocentesis to obtain an amniotic fluid sample.

• Simpson et al. (1976) and others have shown fewer complications associated with amniocentesis when a smaller 20 or 21 gauge needle is used.

• Simpson et al. (1976) also have shown significantly fewer complications (2.8% versus 7.3%) associated with amniocentesis when it is performed at or after 16 weeks gestation.

4. Discussion

Assessments of the technologies used in NTD screening should include two levels of analysis: the individual technologies and the complete screening protocol. We found that the literature is dominated by studies of the individual technologies. The papers that analyze the screening protocol emphasize diagnostic outcomes. There is less analysis of factors such as interactions between tests, a broad range of patient outcomes, and the clinical course of patients who did not follow the usual screening protocol.

In this analysis, we compare the literature on technologies used in prenatal screening for NTDs to the standards of technology assessment. The discussion focuses on gaps in the literature, but it should be noted that there is a large and growing body of pertinent scientific knowledge. The volume and quality of work are impressive and while we focus on problem areas, we do not intend to suggest that there are not at least as many areas of strength and scientific rigor.

In general, the literature on the technologies used in prenatal NTD screening provides uneven information. Some of the gaps are especially compelling, and are identified below.

Gaps in information about MSAFP

• New mathematical models for interpreting MSAFP values make use of maternal factors such as weight and medical history, and fetal factors such as gestational age. The effectiveness of MSAFP would change if these kinds of data were generally available.

• Pilot studies of NTD screening indicate that a significant number of women do not participate in MSAFP screening. Who makes these choices, why, and what happens to those pregnancies? To understand the effectiveness of MSAFP, we will need to know more about the outcomes for all pregnant women. The state of California recently mandated that MSAFP be offered to all pregnant women, thus creating an opportunity to begin to answer these questions.

Gaps in information about ultrasonography

• The Consensus group on diagnostic ultrasonography in pregnancy indicated that it is essential to continue to evaluate safety. The group also raised issues regarding standards for equipment and operator training. The way in which these issues are resolved will affect efficacy and effectiveness as well.

• The appropriate use of ultrasonographic findings remains undetermined. Reports indicate that confidence in the findings varies among clinicians, which leaves some uncertainty about the diagnostic impact of ultrasonography. Will ultrasonography replace other tests such as amniocentesis? Under what conditions? Should this procedure be considered the final test?

Gaps in information about amniocentesis for AF-AFP measurement and AChE assay

• Recent findings suggest methods for reducing complications of amniocentesis. Should further large-scale studies be performed to determine the optimal conditions for amniocentesis? Are there other factors, such as anxiety or stress, that affect the probability of untoward effects?

• The accuracy of AF-AFP measurement is dependent on the quality of the sample of amniotic fluid, but even with high quality samples, the methods for calibrating the test results and establishing cutoffs for abnormal values present problems similar to those found in MSAFP testing. The literature describes the role of AChE in improving diagnostic accuracy, but this test was not included in the pilot NTD screening program reports included in this review. Would the improved diagnostic power of AChE be seen in large-scale applications?

• Should AF-AFP and AChE be used as the final step in testing, or should Stage II ultrasonography become the next step? We found little analysis of the relative costs and benefits to be expected if ultrasonography was used to confirm AFP and AChE findings.

Gaps in information about screening program

• The depth and breadth of information about all of these screening tests taken together, as a screening program, are limited. This information can only be gained through pilot screening programs that assess the effectiveness of the entire battery of tests. The final assessment of these technologies rests on the data regarding their joint performance. We found several crucial gaps in such data.

• We found little discussion or analysis of the availability of the screening tests. There was even less discussion of specific issues, such as access to the most appropriate equipment and operators, supportive services, and the resources that make a range of parental choices truly possible.

• We found little discussion of the effects of screening on two groups: women who do not follow the usual screening protocol, and the fetus.

• In one of the pilot studies (Milunsky and Alpert, 1984), diagnostic accuracy of the screening protocol was enhanced by use of a coordinated system of expert obstetricians, clinical geneticists, and experienced laboratory staff and ultrasonographers. However, we found little analysis of how these factors should be used in analyses of the value of NTD screening for a population.

• We found no studies that describe a broad range of costs and benefits to pregnant women experiencing NTD screening, with psychological dimensions being most neglected.

5. Conclusions

This analysis was conducted to illustrate how technology assessment can contribute to policy analysis. It was not intended to reach a conclusion about the safety, efficacy, and effectiveness of the technologies under discussion. Rather, it uses these standards of technology assessment to identify gaps in knowledge. Several gaps that were identified are: the method of choice for calibrating MSAFP and AF-AFP is not yet well established; the outcomes for women who do not participate in MSAFP testing are not well documented; the safety of ultrasonography during pregnancy is not fully confirmed; and the contributions of AChE to large-scale screening are not known. There are also gaps in knowledge about the tests taken together as a screening protocol. For example, there is little analysis of availability and access issues, of the psychological costs and benefits of screening, and of the effects of screening on the fetus and on women when the usual protocol is not followed. This field is characterized by rapid development and ongoing research, therefore, some of these gaps may have been addressed since we completed our analysis.

Technology assessment is used most frequently to examine and refine tests and laboratory procedures. In that case, the standards of efficacy, effectiveness, and safety are goals to be achieved. Here, we used the standards as the benchmarks of well-balanced and comprehensive knowledge. This approach to technology assessment offers a unique opportunity to see the field as a whole. The findings are important because they describe the quality of knowledge about the technologies. For example, if the literature about the technologies used in prenatal NTD screening fully addressed the standards of efficacy, effectiveness, and safety, it would provide a sound basis for determining how best to use the technologies. When the basis is not as sound, it is important to know where the gaps are. This kind of information is especially useful to health care professionals and state and federal policymakers responsible for determining the testing protocols that should be made available to all pregnant women.

For example, the state of California has recently mandated that all pregnant women be offered the option of MSAFP screening. To implement such a mass screening program effectively, the health care professionals in California need the most up-to-date information on the assessment of the MSAFP test, and the other procedures that follow. A review of what is known through published studies forms one basis for this knowledge and can be used as background material for reaching consensus by groups of experts brought together by the National Institutes of Health, or others, such as individual state departments of health.

Technology assessment through literature review cannot answer all of the questions about applications of medical technology, but the questions that are answered and the gaps in knowledge that are identified provide valuable information.

6. Footnotes

[1]Completed in 1984.
[2]The disorder and the technologies are described in Part I.
[3]Adapted from Fineberg et al. (1977) and Banta et al. (1981)
[4]The FDA assumed 1-2 per 1,000 live births as the incidence of NTDs.

7. References

Adams, M.J., Windham, G.C., James, L.M., Greenberg, F., Clayton-Hopkins, J.A., Reimer, C.B., and Oakley, G.P. Clinical interpretation of maternal serum alpha-fetoprotein concentrations. *American Journal of Obstetrics and Gynecology*, 1984, *148*, 241-254.

American College of Obstetricians and Gynecologists (ACOG). Diagnostic ultrasound in obstetrics and gynecology. *ACOG Technical Bulletin*, No. 63. Washington, DC, 1981.

American College of Obstetricians and Gynecologists (ACOG). Prenatal detection of neural tube defects. *ACOG Technical Bulletin*, No. 67. Washington, DC, 1982.

Amniotic fluid acetylcholinesterase electrophoresis as a secondary test in the diagnosis of anencephaly and open spina bifida in early pregnancy: Report of the Collaborative Acetylcholinesterase Study. *Lancet*, 1981, *2*, 321-324.

Banta, H.D., Behney, C.J., and Willems, J.S. *Toward rational technology in medicine*. New York: Springer Publishing Company, 1981.

Benacerraf, B.R. and Frigoletto, F.D. Amniocentesis under continuous ultrasound guidance: A series of 232 cases. Unpublished manuscript, Brigham and Women's Hospital, Boston, MA. 1983.

Bennett, M.J., Little, G., Dewhurst, J., and Chamberlain, G. Predictive value of ultrasound measurement in early pregnancy: A randomized trial. *British Journal of Obstetrics and Gynaecology*, 1982, *89*, 348-351.

Beuamah, P.K., Evans, L., and Ward, A.M. Amniotic fluid acetylcholinesterase isoenzyme patterns in the diagnosis of neural tube defects. *Clinica Chimica Acta*, 1980, *103*, 146-151.

Brock, D. J. H. Impact of maternal serum alpha-fetoprotein screening on antenatal diagnosis. *British Medical Journal*, 1982, *285*, 365-367.

Brock, D.J.H. Neural tube defects and alpha-fetoprotein: An international perspective. In: M. Kaback (Ed.) *Genetic issues in pediatric and obstetric practice*. Chicago: Year Book Medical Publishers, 1981.

Brock, D.J.H. Ultrasound in detection of neural tube defects. *Lancet*, 1983, *2*, 1251-1252.

Brock, D.J.H., Barron, L., Duncan, P., Scrimgeour, J.B., and Watt, M. Significance of elevated mid-trimester maternal plasma alpha-fetoprotein values. *Lancet*, 1979, 1281-1282.

Brock, D.J.H., Barron, L., Watt, M., Scrimgeour, J.B., and Keay, A.J. Maternal plasma alpha-fetoprotein and low birthweight: A prospective study throughout pregnancy. *British Journal of Obstetrics and Gynaecology*, 1982, *89*, 348-351.

Brock, D.J.H. and Hayward, C. Gel electrophoresis of amniotic fluid acetylcholinesterase as an aid to the prenatal diagnosis of fetal defects. *Clinica Chimica Acta*, 1980, *108*, 135-141.

Brock, D.J.H. and Sutcliffe, R.G. Alpha-fetoprotein in the antenatal diagnosis of anencephaly and spina bifida. *Lancet*, 1972, *2*, 197-9.

Campbell, S. Early prenatal diagnosis of neural tube defects by ultrasound. *Clinical Obstetrics and Gynecology*, 1977, *20*, 351-359.

Crandall, B.F., Lebherz, T.B., and Freihube, R. Neural tube defects: Maternal serum screening and prenatal diagnosis. *Pediatric Clinics of North America*, 1978, *25*, 619-629.

Dale, G., Archibald, A., Bonham, J.R., and Lowdon, P. Diagnosis of neural tube defects by estimation of amniotic fluid acetylcholinesterase. *British Journal of Obstetrics and Gynaecology*, 1981, *88*, 120-125.

Department of Health and Human Services (DHHS). Food and Drug Administration, Public Health Service and Health Care Financing Administration. Alpha-fetoprotein test kits: Proposed restrictions and additional quality control and testing requirements. *Federal Register*, November 7, 1980, *45*, 74158-74176.

Department of Health and Human Services. *Diagnostic ultrasound imaging in pregnancy: Report of a consensus conference*. Washington: Superintendent of Documents, 1984 (NIH Publication No. 84-667).

Epley, S.L., Hanson, J.W., and Cruikshank, D.P. Fetal injury with midtrimester diagnostic amniocentesis. *Obstetrics and Gynecology*, 1979, *53*, 77-80.

Ferguson-Smith, M.A. Concluding remarks. In Jan-Diether Murken (Ed.), *Prenatal Diagnosis*. Stuttgart: Ferdinand Enke Publishers, 1979.

Fineberg, H.V., Bauman, R., and Sosman, M. Computerized cranial tomography: Effect on diagnostic and therapeutic plans. *Journal of the American Medical Association*, 1977, *238*, 224-227.

Fletcher, J. and Evans, M.I. Maternal bonding in early fetal ultrasound examinations. *New England Journal of Medicine*, 1983, *308*, 392-393.

Gardner, S., Burton, B.K., and Johnson, A.M. Maternal serum alpha-fetoprotein screening: A report of the Forsyth County Project. *American Journal of Obstetrics and Gynecology*, 1981, *140*, 250-253.

Golbus, M.S., Loughman, W.D., Epstein, C.J., Halbasch, G., Stephens, J.D., and Hall, B.D. Prenatal genetic diagnosis in 3000 amniocenteses. *New England Journal of Medicine*, 1979, *300*, 157-163.

Goldberg, M.F. and Oakley, G.P. Prenatal screening for anencephaly-spina bifida: Some epidemiological projections for a national program. In Porter, I.H. and Hook, E.B. (Eds.) *Service and education in medical genetics*. New York: Academic Press, 1979.

Greenberg, F., James, L.M. and Oakley, G.P. Estimates of birth prevalence rates of spina bifida in the United States from computer generated maps. *American Journal of Obstetrics and Gynecology*, 1983, *145*, 570-573.

Haddow, J.E., Morin, M.E., Holman, M.S., and Miller, W.A. Acetylcholinesterase and fetal malformations: Modified qualitative technique for diagnosis of neural tube defects. *Clinical Chemistry*, 1981, *27*, 61-63.

Hamburg, D.A. Towards more judicious use of biomedical technology in health care. In: *Evaluating medical technologies in clinical use*. (Conference Summary). Washington, DC: National Academy Press, 1981.

Harris, R. and Read, A.P. New uncertainties in prenatal screening for neural tube defects. *British Medical Journal*, 1981, *282*, 1416-1418.

Hobbins, J.C., Venus, I., Tortora, M., Mayden, L., and Mahoney, M.J. Stage II ultrasound examination for the diagnosis of fetal abnormalities with an elevated amniotic fluid alpha-fetoprotein concentration. *American Journal of Obstetrics and Gynecology*, 1982, *142*, 1026-1029.

Holtzman, N.A., Leonard, C.O., and Farfel, M.R. Issues in antenatal and neonatal screening and surveillance for hereditary and congenital disorders. *American Review of Public Health*, 1981, *2*, 219-251.

Layde, P.M., von Allmen, S.D., and Oakley, G.P., Jr. Maternal serum alpha-fetoprotein screening: A cost-benefit analysis. *American Journal of Public Health*, 1979, *69*, 566-573.

Lele, A.S., Carmody, P.J., Hurd, M.E., and O'Leary, J.A. Fetomaternal bleeding following diagnostic amniocentesis. *Obstetrics and Gynecology*, 1982, *60*, 60-64.

Leonard, C.O. Serum AFP screening for neural tube defects. *Clinical Obstetrics and Gynecology*, 1981, *24*, 1121-1132.

Macri, J.N., Haddow, J.E., and Weiss, R.R. Screening for neural tube defects in the United States. A summary of the Scarborough Conference. *American Journal of Obstetrics and Gynecology*, January 15, 1979, *133*, 119-125.

Macri, J.N., Weiss, R.R., and Libster, B. Maternal serum alpha-fetoprotein screening for neural tube defects: Structure and organization. In Porter, I.H. and Hook, E.B. (Eds.) *Service and education in medical genetics*. New York: Academic Press, 1979.

Mennuti, M.T., Brummond, W., Crombleholme, W.R., Schwarz, R.H., and Arvan, D.A. Fetal-maternal bleeding associated with genetic amniocentesis. *Obstetrics and Gynecology*, 1980, *55*, 48-54.

Milunsky, A. and Alpert, E. Results and benefits of a maternal serum alpha-fetoprotein screening program. *Journal of the American Medical Association*, 1984, *252*, 1438-1442.

Milunsky, A. and Sapirstein, V.S. Prenatal diagnosis of open neural tube defects using the amniotic fluid acetylcholinesterase assay. *Obstetrics and Gynecology*, 1982, *59*, 1-5.

National Institute of Child Health and Human Development (NICHHD). National Registry for Amniocentesis Study Group. Midtrimester amniocentesis for prenatal diagnosis: Safety and accuracy. *Journal of the American Medical Association*, 1976, *236*, 1471-1476.

National Institute of Child Health and Human Development (NICHHD). *Antenatal diagnosis: Report of Consensus Conference*. 1979.

Read, A.P., Fennell, S.J., Donnai, D., and Harris, R. Amniotic fluid acetylcholinesterase: A retrospective and prospective study of the qualitative method. *British Journal of Obstetrics and Gynaecology*, 1982, *89*, 218-221.

Reading, A.E. and Cox, D.N. The effects of ultrasound examination on maternal anxiety levels. *Journal of Behavioral Medicine*, 1982, *5*, 237-247.

Roberts, C.J., Hibbard, B.M., Roberts, E.E., Evans, K.T., Laurence, K.M. and Robertson, I.B. Diagnostic effectiveness of ultrasound in detection of neural tube defects. *Lancet*, *1*, 1983, 1068-1069.

Seller, M.J. and Cole, K.J. Polyacrylamide gel electrophoresis of amniotic fluid acetylcholinesterase: A good prenatal test for neural tube defects. *British Journal of Obstetrics and Gynaecology*, 1980, *87*, 1103-1108.

Simpson, N.E., Dallaire, L., Miller, J.R., Siminovich, L., Hamerton, J.L., Miller, J. and McKeen, C. Prenatal diagnosis of genetic disease in Canada: Report of a collaborative study. *Canadian Medical Association Journal*, 1976, *115*, 739-746.

Smith, A.F. Amniotic fluid acetylcholinesterase assay and the antenatal detection of neural tube defects. *Clinica Chimica Acta*, 1982, *123*, 1-9.

Sowers, S.G. and Burton, B.K. The clinical significance of low maternal serum alpha-fetoprotein in obstetric practice. *Birth defects: Original article series*, 1982, *18*, 181-184.

UK Collaborative Study. Survival of infants with open spina bifida in relation to maternal serum alpha-fetoprotein level. *British Journal of Obstetrics and Gynaecology*, 1982, *89*, 3-7.

Varma, T.R. Amniocentesis in early pregnancy using free-hand needle technique under ultrasonic control. *International Journal of Gynecology and Obstetrics*, 1981, *19*, 145-54.

Verp, M.S. and Gerbie, A.B. Amniocentesis for prenatal diagnosis. *Clincial Obstetrics and Gynecology*, 1981, *24*, 1007-1021.

Wald, N.J. and Cuckle, H.S. Amniotic fluid acetylcholinesterase electrophoresis as a secondary test in the diagnosis of anencephaly and open spina bifida in early pregnancy. *Lancet*, 1981, *2*, 321-324.

Watson, D., Pow, M., Ellam, A., and Costeloe, K. Prevention of neural tube defects in an urban health district. *Journal of Epidemiology and Community Health*, 1983, *37*, 221-225.

Wortman, P.M. and Saxe, L. Assessment of medical technology: Methodological considerations. In *Assessing the efficacy and safety of medical technologies*. (Office of Technology Assessment). U.S. Government Printing Office, No. 052-003-00593-0, 1978.

B. Prenatal Screening for Neural Tube Defects: Use of Decision Analysis

Barbara J. McNeil, M.D., Ph.D.
Stephen G. Pauker, M.D. *

Public policy makers and physicians are frequently required to make decisions in the presence of incomplete data. Decision analysis is an approach, actually a set of modeling techniques, that provides insight into the tradeoffs inherent in the decision at hand. Decision analysis is a formal and explicit way of answering questions like, "What is the most cost-effective approach to screening small children for lead poisoning?" Or, "What is the extra cost per extra quality-adjusted life-year gained from introducing diagnostic test 'X' or treatment 'Y'?"

In the public policy arena, the most valuable feature of decision analysis is its explicit nature. The problem and its alternatives must be formulated explicitly, data on all events must be quantified to the extent possible, and, finally, values (societal or individual) must be placed on the resulting outcomes. The impact of disagreements about the data can be discussed at the hands of sensitivity analyses.

In this chapter we will review the role of decision analysis in prenatal disease by discussing a recent example done on the problem of whether or not to institute a screening program for neural tube defects (NTDs). We will also formulate the approach that is appropriate for analyzing a more contemporary problem—the value of routine second trimester ultrasonographic screening examinations in pregnant women. The reader is directed to several references for further information in this area (Raiffa, 1970; Keeney and Raiffa, 1976; Weinstein et al., 1980).

1. The Alpha-Fetoprotein Problem

Consider the potential value of instituting a screening program in the United States for neural tube defects based on assay of maternal serum for alpha-fetoprotein (AFP). Use of decision analysis to help determine the value of such a program first requires the creation of a model giving the alternatives. Figure 1 illustrates one model for this purpose (Pauker et al., 1981). In this diagram, points of decision ("decision nodes") are depicted by squares, whereas outcomes occurring by chance ("chance nodes") are depicted by circles.

According to this tree the alternatives involve a decision between screening (upper branch) and no screening (lower branch). If screening is undertaken and is normal, the fetus is presumed to be at low risk for having an NTD. If the screening is abnormal, it is repeated and ultrasonography is recommended if the second test is also abnormal. The second decision node of the upper branch indicates that the patient can either refuse ultrasonography or not. In the latter case, the examination will indicate an explanation for the abnormal AFP level (e.g., by showing twins), will show the presence of a NTD, or will not give a satisfactory explanation for the

---

* From the Departments of Radiology and Preventive Medicine and Clinical Epidemiology, Harvard Medical School and Brigham and Women's Hospital and the Division of Clinical Decision Making, Department of Medicine, New England Medical Center, Boston.

Figure 1
Decision Tree for Prenatal NTD Screening

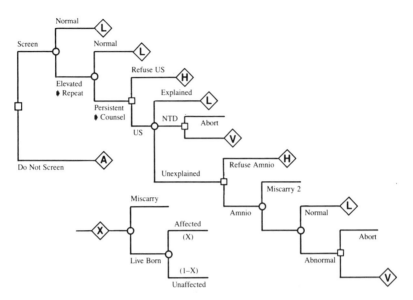

Decision tree for the alpha-fetoprotein decision. The main tree is shown in the top part of the figure; the subtree with X in the diamond denotes the outcomes of pregnancy and is depicted in the lower portion of the figure. Each reference to the subtree is denoted by a diamond. The letter within the diamond refers to the risk of an affected fetus: A for average risk, L for lower than average risk, H for high risk, and V for very high risk. These risks were calculated using Bayes rule (Weinstein et. al., 1980) NTD = neural tube defect; AMNIO = amniocentesis; ABORT = elective abortion; MISCARRY 2 = miscarriage secondary to amniocentesis.

Reproduced with permission from *Ann Rev Public Health* 1984, 5:141.

abnormal AFP. These latter two alternatives are associated with choices on the part of the patient, as shown in the figure. As the reader follows the consequences resulting from each of these decisions, he or she will always end at a common subtree, shown as a diamond, or at an abortion, or at a miscarriage.

These subtrees at eight points of the "screen" strategy and at one point of the "no screen" strategy all have the same structure shown at the bottom of the figure. As a result of the interventions up to this point in the tree a patient can either miscarry or proceed through a pregnancy and have a child with or without an NTD. The chances of these outcomes differ at varying points in the decision tree depending upon the sequence of diagnostic data leading to that point. For example, the likelihood would be high (H) after two abnormal AFP determinations not explained by another cause but low (L) after a single normal serum test.

In order to determine the relative values of the "screen" and "no screen" strategies in the above decision tree it is necessary to attach *probability* estimates at each of the chance nodes. For example, "how often will ultrasonography reveal an error in the estimated gestational age or the presence of twins in women with two elevated

AFP levels?" "What is the excess miscarriage rate for women having second trimester amniocentesis?" It is also necessary in this analysis to attach values or *utilities* to the four possible outcomes occurring in this situation: parents' attitudes towards an accidental miscarriage resulting from amniocentesis; their attitudes toward an elective abortion; and their attitudes toward the birth of a child affected with a neural tube defect. The birth of a healthy child is assumed to be the best outcome. The third step in the process involves serial multiplication of probabilities times utilities and addition of these products so that the expected utility of the two strategies can be compared.

Probabilistic data are straightforward to obtain, at least conceptually. For the AFP problem, data from Great Britain and recent U.S. studies are applicable. They would answer the above questions as follows: 50% of women will have an explanation for two abnormal AFP levels. The excess miscarriage rate from amniocentesis is probably about 0.5%.

Utility data, on the other hand, are more difficult to obtain and must nearly always be obtained as part of the analysis in question. There are no "utility data banks" to help the analyst. Utility assessments require that attitudes for the conditions under study be placed on a scale from zero to 100, in this case zero implying the birth of a normal child and 100 the birth of a child with a neural tube defect. The value of another outcome, for example an abortion, is obtained by responses to questions such as, "At what chance of a pregnancy's producing a severely deformed child would you prefer elective abortion to the risk of having a live-born child affected with a neural tube defect?" The minimum chance at which they would still prefer abortion is used as a measure of the burden of abortion relative to the burden of an affected child. An analogous question is required to assess the burden of a miscarriage induced by amniocentesis. A recent article by Christensen-Szalanski (1984) may be of interest to readers concerned about the stability of such utility assessments over time.

Fixed values of each of the probabilities and utilities give expected utilities for the "screen" and "no screen" strategies. In this case, the decision problem was formulated as one for society: should the United States institute a screening program? It was not one for an individual patient: should I, as a pregnant woman, have a serum AFP test? Thus, the analysis becomes more complex and varies with the distribution of values in the society for the possible outcomes (miscarriage, abortion, child with an NTD). This distribution influences the extent to which the population being considered would benefit by having the serum screen introduced so that subsequent options are possible. Figure 2 shows such a distribution of results obtained for the burden of an elective abortion for a sample of prospective parents in Boston. The reader is referred to the original article (Pauker et al., 1981) for a further discussion of the details of this analysis.

2. The Value of Screening Ultrasonographic Examinations

For the detection of fetal abnormalities, we are considering the value of routine screening ultrasonographic examinations performed between 16 and 20 weeks. We are assuming that all abnormal ultrasonographic examinations are repeated to confirm any abnormality seen. The decision tree for this problem is considerably more complex than for the AFP problem. In the AFP tree there is only a single target abnormality—a fetus with a neural tube defect. In the tree involving the value of screening ultrasonographic examinations a variety of defects are relevant (Table 1).

Figure 2

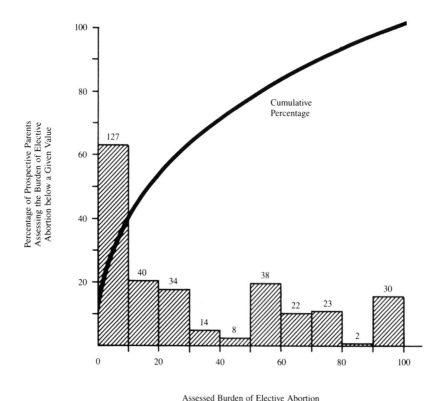

Assessed Burden of Elective Abortion
Percentage of Burden of Affected Child

Distribution of attitudes toward elective abortion of 338 prospective parents seeking genetic counseling. Horizontal axis displays the burden of elective abortion on a scale in which zero denotes no burden and where 100 is the burden of an affected child. The vertical axis denotes the percentage of prospective parents having each attitude shown in the bar graph. The solid curve summarizes the cumulative distribution.

The abnormalities of most concern in this analysis are: hydrocephalus, meningo-myelocele, anencephaly, genitourinary abnormalities, musculoskeletal (e.g., limb reduction) abnormalities, gastroschisis, and a child with multiple congenital abnormalities. The complexity of a *simultaneous* search for these abnormalities (with a single screening examination) has been addressed (Lau et al., 1984). Although such a simultaneous approach prevents undervaluing the diagnostic test under consideration, for reasons of simplicity of explication here, we have assumed a search for

Table 1

Fetal abnormalities potentially detectable on ultrasonographic examination.

Nonspecific findings. The most common of these is an abnormal quantity of amniotic fluid, caused by CNS abnormalities, GI tract obstructions, and some renal abnormalities.

- Cranial abnormalities. Anencephaly and hydrocephalus are the most common.
- Spinal abnormalities. The detection of spina bifida is difficult but possible; for myelomeningoceles ease of detection is roughly proportional to size.
- Chest abnormalities. Diaphragmatic hernias and chest wall abnormalities may be detected in the second trimester. Recent reports document the identification of heart valves and chambers by ultrasonography but this capability is not yet advanced sufficiently to diagnose prospectively fetal cardiac abnormalities.
- Abdominal abnormalities. Omphalocele and gastroschisis can be detected in the second trimester and gastrointestinal atresias and obstructions can frequently be identified. Urinary tract abnormalities can also be detected.
- Disorders of the extremities. A variety of fetal anomalies affect limb length. Standards of normal limb lengths have been developed for different gestational ages and are updated as more information becomes available.
- Multisystem anomalies. All of the above findings may occur in fetuses with multiple congenital anomalies.

only one abnormality, hydrocephalus. Figure 3 shows the decision tree for this purpose.

In this tree the first decision node indicates the fundamental decision—do an ultrasonography or not. In both cases the fetus may or may not have hydrocephalus at a rate determined by the underlying prevalence in the population (about 10 per 10,000). If no ultrasonography is performed (upper branch), no additional information exists about the probability of a normal versus a deformed fetus, and the analyst moves right on to a subtree called "Prognosis." This indicates that sometime during the pregnancy a miscarriage can occur or not. If it does not, the outcomes are: stillborn, liveborn with perinatal death, liveborn without hydrocephalus, liveborn with hydrocephalus and minor disability, liveborn with hydrocephalus and major disability.

If ultrasonography is performed, additional information on the probability of hydrocephalus is available. If two tests are obtained and are positive (these can be either true positives or false positives), then the patient usually proceeds to an additional workup (subtree "Next Step"). If the ultrasonography is negative (these can be either true negatives or false negatives), then the subtree "Prognosis" is relevant. For suspected hydrocephalus, the next confirming step is amniocentesis with measurement of amniotic AFP levels. The procedure can lead to a miscarriage or not. In the latter case, if the test results are positive, there is a possibility that the parents will seek a therapeutic abortion.

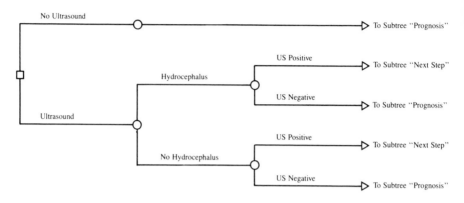

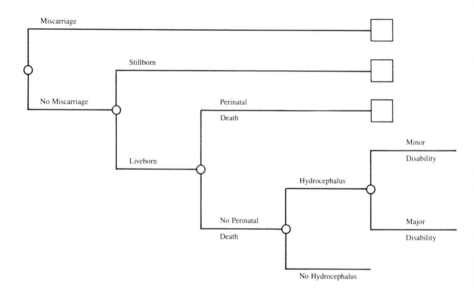

62

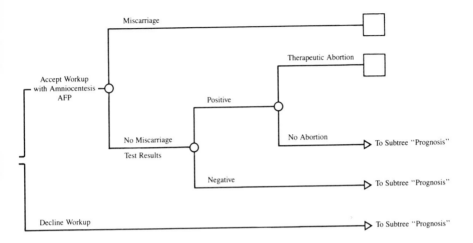

Decision tree and subtrees for ultrasonography (US) versus no ultrasonographic decision. Subtree "Next Step" indicates the workup required when two ultrasonographic examination are abnormal and suggest that hydrocephalus is present. Subtree "Prognosis" indicates the outcomes possible if no interventions are performed. The rectangles at the end of each branch indicate the end of the options for the tree at that point and are the outcomes for which utility values are needed.

In this analysis, many probabilities must be obtained. In the initial tree, for example, it is necessary to have information about the prevalence of hydrocephalus and the sensitivity and specificity of ultrasonography in its detection. In subtree "Next Step" the analyst must know how often amniocentesis induces a miscarriage. In subtree "Prognosis" the proportion of liveborns afflicted with minor or major sequelae of hydrocephalus must be known.

In terms of utilities, the overall approach is similar to that shown in the AFP tree, but, in this case, a greater spectrum of outcomes exists: miscarriage, miscarriage induced by amniocentesis, therapeutic abortion, stillborn child, perinatal death, child with minor abnormalities, or child with major abnormalities. Apart from these health outcomes a complete decision analysis would also show the financial implications of the two strategies.

For the ultrasonographic problem some of the results can be summarized as follows. With routine screening for any of the starred abnormalities shown in Table 1, the major effect of ultrasonography is the prevention of the birth of some defective fetuses as well as the movement of financially expensive losses in the perinatal period to less expensive therapeutic abortions. "Second trimester ultrasound resulted in an average excess cost of $67 per pregnancy and 27 therapeutic abortions per 10,000 pregnancies. The 27 therapeutic abortions performed were the results of averting 11 spontaneous abortions, 9 affected infants, and 7 perinatal deaths. The number of normal infants aborted due to false positive results was less than 3 per 100 million pregnancies" (Lau et al., 1984).

Even more interesting results occur when maternal serum AFP screening and a routine second trimester ultrasonographic examination are viewed together (Lau et al., 1984). If the maternal serum AFP is not elevated, then the chance of an NTD (the most common type of anomaly detected by ultrasonographic screening) is lowered sufficiently to make screening ultrasonography no longer cost-effective.

3. Conclusions

Decision analysis is an approach which forces public policy analysts acting in behalf of society, or physicians acting in behalf of their patients, to make explicit all factors they are considering for the choice at hand. They must, in addition, attach quantitative estimates to these factors. Ideally, such estimates should be based on objective data. Unfortunately, objective data are usually scarce, particularly for pressing new situations, and analysts must frequently rely on subjective estimates. Such estimates may be biased (Tversky and Kahneman, 1974, 1981; McNeil et al., 1982), but with appropriate sensitivity analyses performed using ranges of estimates, it is possible to determine the robustness of the conclusion. Such analyses may also identify the factor dominating the final recommendation. For example, in the ultrasonographic problem, the most significant variable could be the specificity of ultrasonography, the sensitivity of ultrasonography, or perhaps the attitudes of society towards therapeutic abortion.

Although decision analyses can be time consuming and frustrating because of difficulties in obtaining reliable data, they appear to be increasing in the medical field. Recently, as part of several Consensus Development Conferences sponsored by the National Institutes of Health, decision analyses have been done simultaneously with the more conventional "expert consensus" approach. We believe that this trend will continue and will extend to other organizations. Because of society's current concern with its limited resources for health, it will become increasingly important for us to answer a series of "what if" questions in a timely fashion. Advances in molecular genetics suggest that questions involving prenatal diagnosis and *in utero* therapy may benefit most from this technique.

Acknowledgments

We are grateful for the help of the Working Group on Disease Prevention of the Division of Health Policy, Research and Education, Harvard University for their comments during preparation of this review. We are also indebted to the Office of Medical Applications of Research of the National Institutes of Health for providing us with insight in the details of the ultrasonographic problem, gained as a result of a consensus conference on this subject.

4. References

Christensen-Szalanski, J.J. Discount functions and the measurement of patients' values: Women's decisions during childbirth. *Medical Decision Making*, 1984, *4*, 47-58.

Keeney, R. and Raiffa, H. *Decisions with multiple objectives: Preference and tradeoff value tradeoffs*. New York: Wiley, 1976.

Lau, J., Frigoletto, F., McNeil B.J., Zarin, D.A., and Pauker, S.G. Diagnostic ultrasound in prenatal screening for congenital abnormalities. *Medical Decision Making, 1984, 4,* 545.

Lau, J. and Pauker, S.G. The use of diagnostic ultrasound imaging in pregnancy. NIH Consensus Development Conference Decision Analysis Project, February 6-8, 1984, Bethesda, Maryland.

McNeil, B.J., Pauker, S.G., Sox, H.C., and Tversky, A. On the elicitation of preferences for alternative therapies. *New England Journal of Medicine*, 1982, *306*, 1259-1262.

Pauker, S.G., Pauker, S.P. and McNeil, B.J. The effect of private attitudes on public policy: Prenatal screening for neural tube defects as a prototype. *Medical Decision Making*, 1981, *1*, 103-114.

Raiffa, H. *Decision analysis. Introductory analysis on choices under uncertainty*. Reading, Mass.: Addison-Wesley, 1970.

Tversky, A. and Kahneman, D. Judgment under uncertainty: Heuristics and biases. *Science*, 1974, *185*, 1124-1131.

Tversky, A. and Kahneman, D. The framing of decisions and the rationality of choice. *Science*, 1981, *211*, 453-458.

Weinstein, M.C., Fineberg, H.V., Elstein, A.S., Frazier, H.S., Neuhauser, D., Neutra, R.R., and McNeil, B.J. *Clinical decision analysis*. Philadephia: Saunders, 1980.

C. Cost-Effectiveness of Prenatal Screening for Neural Tube Defects

Susan B. Meister, Ph.D., R.N.
Donald S. Shepard, Ph.D.
Richard Zeckhauser, Ph.D.

1. Introduction

Advances in medical technology have now made it possible to diagnose neural tube defects (NTDs) in the second trimester of pregnancy. In the United States in recent years, this condition has affected 1 to 2 per 1,000 live births. An infant born with an NTD may die within a few days, may be only mildly impaired, or may be severely disabled, with required lifetime care estimated to cost $40,000 to $50,000 a year.[1] Beyond any financial expenses borne by society at large, the emotional and economic costs to the parents may be considerable, and the suffering of the child substantial. Neural tube defects are a serious public health concern.

The ability to identify fetuses affected by NTDs is valuable because ameliorative actions might be taken. With future advances in technology, significant therapeutic treatment for the fetus may become feasible. With limited present capabilities, the optimal action for a pregnant woman with an affected fetus will depend on her values and preferences. The preferences of pregnant women provide the underpinnings of this analysis, the basis for our judgments of welfare. They are assumed to reflect the preferences of potential fathers and other involved parties, and to incorporate adequate consideration of the welfare of the fetus or future child.

There are two major options for a pregnant woman whose fetus is identified as affected with an NTD. She could abort, or she could prepare for the affected child's birth. If abortion is chosen, the costs savings to the health care system are substantial. The emotional impact on the parents and their assessment of the savings in the child's suffering are more difficult to quantify but are presumably positive, since abortion is freely chosen. For women who would not abort, identification of an NTD would make it possible to secure counseling and, more important, to prepare for delivery in specialized facilities where immediate surgery might limit the extent of the infant's disability.

Until now, because the condition is relatively rare and the sequence of tests for it only recently developed, screening for NTDs during pregnancy has been limited. The California legislature, however, mandated a program effective April 1986 to offer NTD testing to all pregnant women in the state, with costs to be borne by the

Susan Meister's and Donald Shepard's research was supported, in part, by grant #7196 to Harvard University from the Robert Wood Johnson Foundation. Shepard's research was also supported, in part, by the Institute for Health Research, a joint program of the Harvard Community Health Plan and Harvard University. Richard Zeckhauser's research was supported by the National Institute for Research Advancement (Japan). A much earlier related paper was presented at Ethical Issues of Perinatal Medicine, Mead Johnson Symposium on Perinatal and Developmental Medicine No. 24, which was held in Vail, Colorado, June 10–14, 1984. It was distributed as Shepard, Meister, and Zeckhauser (1985).

individual patient, her health maintenance organization, or Medi-Cal (Medicaid), the government insurance program for the poor (Propper, 1986). The total costs of such an inclusive program will be substantial. In contrast to Down syndrome, neural tube defects are equally likely to occur in women of all ages. Thus, a screening program must cover the entire range of pregnant women.[2] The costs and health benefits of such a program are quantified in this paper (though benefits are not assigned a dollar value). These assessments are the vital ingredients for a cost-effectiveness analysis, which helps to decide whether a program of prenatal screening for neural tube defects is worthwhile. Our analysis should help to illustrate the potential contributions of such methods.

Several cost-benefit and cost-effectiveness studies of prenatal screening for spina bifida have been reported from the United States (Layde et al., 1979), Canada (Sadovnick and Baird, 1983), South Africa (Grace, 1981), and the United Kingdom (Hibbard et al., 1985; Hagard et al., 1976). The studies found benefit-cost ratios of 2.1 (Layde et al., 1979), 1.8 (Sadovnick and Baird, 1983), and 1.7 (Grace, 1981), indicating that benefits exceed the costs. One U.K. study indicated that the cost of averting the birth of one infant with a neural tube defect who would survive beyond 24 hours as $51,000 (21,400 British pounds) in 1980 prices (Hibbard et al., 1985). While these studies all suggest that a screening program for NTDs would be worthwhile, they fail to address several significant issues.

Overview of this study

This study uses recent data and incorporates several considerations not addressed in earlier analyses. One innovation in this analysis is a recognition that the effects of a testing program will differ radically between two groups: women who would choose to abort an affected fetus and women who would choose to continue the pregnancy, but prepare. We have no reliable estimates of how the population of pregnant women is distributed between these two categories. Indeed many women may not know what their own choice would be until confronted with the necessity to make one. The results of an NTD-testing program in operation would eventually tell us.

Table 1 enumerates the elements of cost-effectiveness applied to this type of problem. Our approach to decision making employs separate utility scales for the two categories of pregnant women. We leave the decision whether to abort or prepare to individuals and assess the costs and benefits that follow from their choices. In essence, each woman in the population is confronted with a decision analysis.

For women who choose abortion, the savings in avoided medical costs for a disabled child are appropriately weighed against the costs of the testing program. For women who choose to go to term with an identified NTD fetus, the relevant benefits are those achieved through advanced planning for birth in a specialized facility. Without introducing further value judgments, there is no valid way to combine results for these two groups into a single cost-benefit or cost-effectiveness assessment.

If separate analyses showed that a testing program is merited for women who would choose to abort but not for women who would carry the pregnancy to term (or vice versa), the appropriate policy decision would have to depend on judgments as to the relative sizes of the two groups or their behavior in practice. For example, women who know they would not abort might refuse a voluntary testing procedure. Given present mores, it would seem unacceptable to limit the program to only those

67

Table 1
Elements of a cost-effectiveness analysis

Element	Issues
Structure	What are the alternatives (decisions)?
	What are the "chance events" (outcomes beyond the control of the decision maker?)
	What is the sequence of decisions and outcomes of chance events becoming known?
Probabilities	What are the initial probabilities of various outcomes?
	How do those probabilities change (become updated) as additional information becomes available?
Costs	Monetary costs
	Nonmonetary costs (e.g., time, discomfort, anxiety, pain)
Utilities	Losses for incorrect decisions
	Create a scale anchored by no loss, and a severe loss (e.g., fail to detect a case of spina bifida)

who would abort, since the "continue to term" group would benefit on net by learning when to prepare.

As discussed in the sections that follow, several other factors complicate the assessment of an NTD testing program. Screening involves a sequence of tests, beginning with a relatively inexpensive maternal blood test and culminating in amniocentesis for those who have had consistently positive test results and for whom ultrasonography is not diagnostic.[3] Amniocentesis requires skilled personnel and costs hundreds of dollars. Some test results are not simply positive or negative, but represent values along a continuous scale. The design of the screening program must determine what cutoffs to use. For example, should the 95th percentile or the 99th percentile level of a marker of NTD (scaled against the values found for unaffected fetuses) be considered a positive result on the first blood test? That choice will influence the diagnostic accuracy of the testing program, its cost, and its effectiveness.

Our analysis relies on empirical data drawn from the medical literature. Although we have used the best numbers available, they are subject to debate, to revision with new findings, or to alteration with improvements in testing technology. We believe, however, that the use of other data sets would not change our conclusions substantially.

Background on neural tube defects

Neural tube defects are congenital abnormalities that occur when the neural tube does not fully close early in the development of a fetus. The most common form of NTD is spina bifida, which occurs when a portion of the spinal column does not close. Resulting disabilities vary widely, depending on the presence, location, and size of a meningomyelocele, a sac containing spinal cord and nerves that protrudes from the infant's back. The most severe forms of spina bifida lead to hydrocephalus (enlargement of the cavities of the brain and accumulation of fluid), severe lower limb paralysis, the absence of bowel and bladder control, recurring urinary infection, mental impairment, and a short life expectancy, often ending in childhood. In less severe cases the child may be able to walk with braces, exercise satisfactory bowel and bladder control, and have little or no mental impairment. Spina bifida occulta, the least severe form, often involves none of the disabilities listed above.

Anencephaly, which comprises roughly 46 percent of the cases of NTD, results from inadequate development of the brain and skull. Affected infants are either stillborn or die within a few days.

2. Elements of the Analysis

Screening for NTDs can provide reasonably accurate information beginning around the sixteenth week of pregnancy. But there are liabilities. The tests, like most medical tests, are not perfectly accurate because they yield both false positive and false negative results. Some NTDs will not be identified, and some women will mistakenly be told that their fetuses are affected when they are actually free of NTDs. Moreover, screening itself may intensify anxiety among those tested, particularly when the first result is positive (suggests that an abnormality may be present), even though the ultimate result may be negative.[4] The program's costs extend beyond the monetary expenditures for testing to include the time and discomfort of patients and their anxiety.

Structure of the screening program

The screening program discussed here consists of a sequence of four tests followed by an action chosen by the woman:
1. Initial determination of maternal serum alpha-fetoprotein (MSAFP).
   (Abnormally high levels of alpha-fetoprotein in a pregnant woman's blood are associated with an NTD in the fetus.)
2. Repeat MSAFP.
3. Ultrasonography, to verify gestational age and to look for NTDs.
4. Amniocentesis to measure alpha-fetoprotein (AFP) in the amniotic fluid.
5. Woman's decision whether to abort, prepare, or merely continue pregnancy.

If either of the first two tests yields a negative result, the screening stops and the fetus is presumed free of NTDs. If ultrasonography reveals that a misjudged gestational age explains the elevated MSAFP, testing stops as well. In some screening programs, if ultrasonography identifies an NTD, screening stops. In this analysis, however, we assumed that these women would be offered amniocentesis. After a positive finding on any test, or if ultrasonography confirms the presumed gestational age, the pregnant woman is offered the next test. If the final test, amniotic fluid AFP, is positive, the woman is informed that her fetus is at very high risk of an NTD. Through counseling she is presented with two major options: termination of pregnancy (abortion) or preparation for the birth of an affected child. She could also choose, however, to continue her pregnancy and not prepared. Each test can be represented as a decision tree like that depicted in Figure 1.

The possible findings at each test represent "chance events." We also consider a woman's choice whether to accept or decline an offered test to be a chance event. On all other choices, we assume that a woman optimizes. Thus, a woman who proceeds through all recommended tests is assumed to take the correct ultimate decision, i.e., abort, prepare, or merely continue pregnancy on the basis of calibrated possibilities of NTDs and her own preferences.

Figure 1
Structure of a Prototypical Screening Program

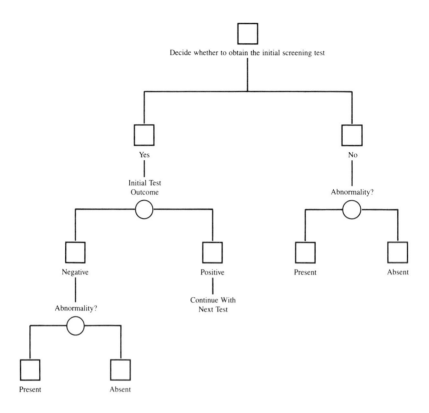

In the design of a testing program, several decisions must be made even if the nature and sequence of tests are clear, such as whether to offer or recommend the initial test, and what cutoff levels to use as positive indicators.

Probabilities

Three types of probabilities must be known or estimated to analyze whether an NTD screening program is desirable: incidence of the conditions among pregnancies, test performance (including interaction among tests), and dropout rates of participants from the program. Our hypothetical population of participants consists of one million pregnant women. They are sixteen weeks pregnant, free of family history of NTDs, receiving prenatal care, and participating in the initial MSAFP screening,

Table 2
Incidence of relevant conditions

Type of Pregnancy	Incidence per Million Pregnancies	Source
A	747	Goldberg and Oakley (1979)
SB	870	Goldberg and Oakley (1979)
Multiple gestation	9,450	National Center for Health Statistics (1982)
Unaffected	988,933	Remainder
All	1,000,000	Total

the blood test that represents the first step in the detection of neural tube defects. An alternative population would be the number of women in an actual geographic area, such as a state, who might participate in a proposed program. While the proportions derived below are important, the absolute size of the cohort was chosen for convenience.

Multiple-gestation pregnancies (e.g., twins) are important because they can produce false positive readings on the MSAFP tests. Although some non-NTD anomalies can also produce false positives, ultrasonography and clinical or other data can usually rule them out. Thus we categorize our cohort of pregnant women according to four types of fetuses: anencephaly (A); spina bifida (SB); unaffected; and unaffected multiple gestation. The numbers of anencephaly, spina bifida, and multiple-gestation pregnancies in this cohort were computed using U.S. incidence data (see Table 2). All other pregnancies were assigned to the "unaffected" category, i.e., no NTDs. Other abnormalities were not considered in this analysis.

Our analysis does not disaggregate the rates of NTDs by race (they are higher for whites) or ethnic group (they are higher for English, Irish, and Welsh ancestry). A screening program focused on high-risk women would be more cost-effective than the program for normal risk analyzed here.

Figures 2 through 5 delineate a flow chart that describes the screening program. Each decision triangle allows the woman to continue the pregnancy as normal, abort, or prepare for the birth of a child with NTD. Table A1 in the Appendix details the sources and methods used to calibrate probabilities and estimate the number of women found at each node. Most of the calculations were performed using a spreadsheet program on a personal computer. The first four columns were the four types of fetuses and the rows were test outcomes and choices about participation. The fifth column shows the total number of women in each group. For groups that have a test, this is the number used in cost calculations. Table A2 in the Appendix provides the formulas for computations, and Table A3 in the Appendix presents the numerical results for the base case.

Figure 2
First MSAFPᵃ

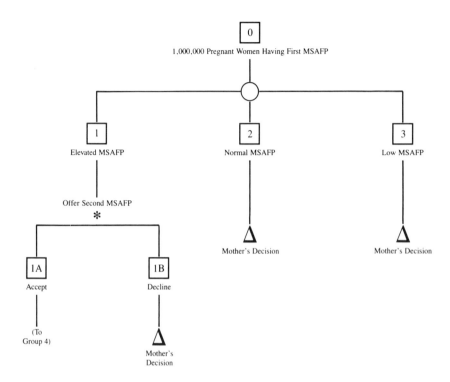

Notes:

ᵃ Circles (○) denote chance events that relate to test outcomes and asterisks (*) relate to choices of participants. Triangles (Δ) denote terminal nodes at which women must decide whether to continue their pregnancy, abort or prepare. SFD denotes spontaneous fetal death.

This Figure describes the outcome of the first MSAFP test. We classified the entire cohort according to type of fetus (anencephaly, spina bifada, unaffected, singletons, multiple gestations); the four subcohorts enter testing as Group 0.

Figure 3
Second MSAFP

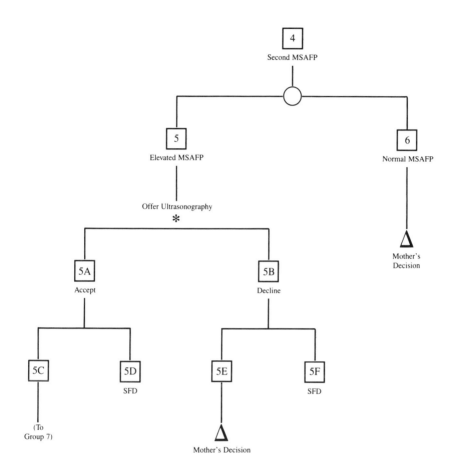

Group 1A from Figure 2 becomes Group 4 in Figure 3, and the second MSAFP reclassifies the group.

Figure 4
Ultrasonography

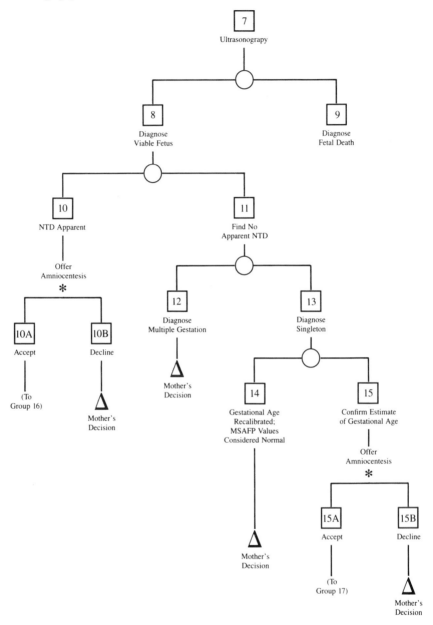

Group 5C from Figure 3 becomes Group 7 in Figure 4; these women have ultrasonographic examinations. Although an ultrasonographer would simultaneously evaluate fetal death, presence of visible NTD, presence of multiple gestation and gestational age, our analytic tree shows each of these findings as a separate node.

Amniocentesis Following Apparent NTD on Ultrasonography

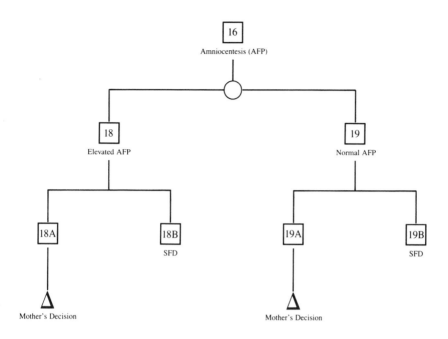

Although the structures of trees in Figures 5A and 5B are identical, we have shown Figure 5 in two sections to clarify that two groups of women are having amniocentesis; the group that had NTDs visualized on ultrasonography (Group 10A, which becomes Group 16); and the group that had essentially negative ultrasonographic findings (Group 15A, which becomes Group 17).

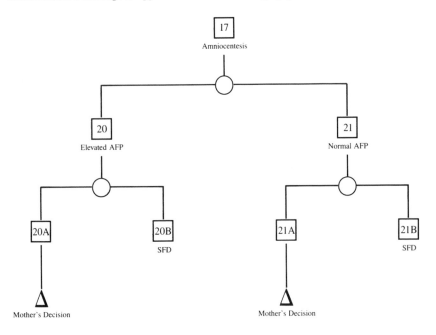

To assess the cost-effectiveness of a screening program, one must classify subjects according to both the true state of their pregnancy (affected or not) and their test results (considered normal or abnormal). For women who complete screening, the test outcome is the result of their final screening test. That is, a woman who has positive results on the first test(s), but a negative reading on her most recent test is classified as having a negative result of screening, indicating that the probability of an NTD is low.

The performance of the first screening test is critical because it separates the entire cohort into three groups, only one of which will have further screening. Measured values of MSAFP fall along a continuum, and there are several possible ways of drawing distinctions between normal and abnormal test results. Our basic analysis uses the 95th percentile as a cutoff; that is, a positive result means the tested woman showed an MSAFP value above that found in 95 percent of women tested in the same laboratory and subsequently confirmed to be unaffected. A more extreme cutoff, the 99th percentile, is sometimes proposed. It would decrease the number of false positives but would also lower the NTD detection rate (Goldberg and Oakely, 1979).

The effectiveness of a screening program depends on how well available tests perform. Performance is usually described in terms of a test's sensitivity (the probability of a positive result for a person with the abnormality), which measures the test's ability to detect an abnormality when it is present and its specificity (the probability of a negative result for a person without the abnormality), which measures the test's ability to rule out an abnormality when it is absent. In this analysis we have applied the sensitivity and specificity values reported by Goldberg and Oakley (1979) (Table 3).

The initial MSAFP screening test has a sensitivity of 88 percent for anencephaly and 78 percent for spina bifida; that is, it identifies between 78 and 88 percent of infants affected with an NTD. Following Goldberg and Oakley (1979), the best available data, we assume that the second MSAFP test uses the same cutoff as the first.

Table 3
Sensitivity and specificity of each test (Percentage)

Test	Sensitivity for:			Specificity
	A	SB	Multiple	(for Unaffected)
First MSAFP	88	78	100	95.0
Second MSAFP[a]	99	99	99	33.3[a]
Ultrasonography	99	0	100	100.0
AFP	90	90	0	99.5

[a] This specificity number is taken from Goldberg and Oakley (1979). They consider two different first tests, one at the 95th percentile, the other at the 99th, but report only a single value for the specificity of their second test.

Table 4
Percentage of pregnancies lost from screening program after each test due to refusal of further testing by mother or spontaneous fetal death[a]

Last Test	Decline Further Testing	Spontaneous Fetal Death
First MSAFP	5.2	8.9
Second MSAFP	1.7	2.1
Ultrasonography	17.6	3.3
AFP (amniocentesis)	—	3.5

[a] Percentages in this table are averages of rates from Gardner, et al., (1981), Goldberg and Oakley (1979), Macri et al., (1979a, 1979b), and Nelson (1983).

Dropout rates from the screening program are the third significant set of probabilities (Table 4). In this analysis, any woman with a positive finding on one screening test who does not accept the next recommended test is considered to have declined further testing (dropped out). A woman who refuses the first test would already be excluded from the cohort. Likely rates of voluntary withdrawal are estimated on the basis of several reports in the literature.

We know of no data indicating the likely behavior of women who fail to continue testing after a positive result. Conceivably they will respond in the same way as women who have been diagnosed as positive after the complete testing program, seeking elective abortion or arranging to deliver in a center particularly well equipped to handle high-risk infants (Propper, 1986). We thought it more reasonable, however, to assume that they will behave like women who never participated in the screening program. Lacking the interest or ability to continue with screening, they were assumed to disregard the test results and take no action. With our assumed utility scales, given the low probability that these women will have an affected fetus, no action (continuing to term) also turns out to be the optimal action. Assuming no action is thus consistent with our general assumption that at the conclusion of screening a woman takes the appropriate action for her, given the probabilities of an affected fetus and her preferences.

There will be further losses from the cohort because at every point through the sequence of tests, some spontaneous fetal deaths (SFD) will occur. Because we did not find a consensus of research establishing differential risks of SFD, this analysis assumes that the rate of SFD is the same for NTD and unaffected fetuses. We assumed screening and follow-up tests have no influence on SFD rates. Amniocentesis, the most risky of the testing procedures, is assumed to carry a 3.5 percent risk of subsequent SFD, about equal to the rate that would occur without that procedure (NICHHD, 1976).[5]

Costs

In our analysis, the monetary costs of screening tests were based on prices charged by a genetic screening service in Southern California in 1983, which proved similar to charges for a public program in Connecticut.[6] These costs, converted to 1984 dollars, are shown in Table 5. Costs, in our analysis, consist of costs for NTD testing and actions during pregnancy. The first screening test (MSAFP) represents 64 percent of the overall cost of the screening program. Although the more sophisticated tests (ultrasonography and amniocentesis for AFP) each cost seven to nine times as much as an MSAFP, they are done on small proportions of the cohort. While an abortion early in the midtrimester costs around $1,200, it would be so rarely performed (925 times for the cohort of 1 million women) that its expected cost is only $1.10 per woman screened.[7] No costs beyond those of screening were included for preparers, since any major additional costs would come after birth.

Table 5

Monetary costs of screening procedures for women who would abort[a]

Test	Unit Cost	Utilization per Woman in Cohort	Cost per Woman in Cohort
First MSAFP	$ 25	1.0000	$25.00
Second MSAFP	25	.0571	1.43
Ultrasonography	180	.0398	7.17
AFP (amniocentesis)	225	.0195	4.39
Abortion	1200	.0009	1.10
Total		1.1174	$39.10

[a] Costs for women who would prepare would be identical except that they do not incur abortion costs. Then, the total cost per woman in the cohort is $38.00

Utilities

In any cost-effectiveness analysis having multiple outcomes, one of the most difficult tasks is to establish utilities for those different treatments and outcomes. The problem is particularly serious for population studies, where meaningful utilities must be based on an accurate understanding of the values to be found in the population.

In the present situation, the probabilities of the highly significant underlying events are not influenced by any decisions made or actions taken. That is, nothing can alter the type of pregnancy: anencephaly, spina bifida, multiple-gestation, or unaffected. Only the treatment that each condition receives is a matter of choice. Thus, the analysis need not consider the base utilities associated with the various possible underlying conditions for the fetus. The mother can choose among medical interventions or treatments such as termination of pregnancy (abortion), planning the delivery in a hospital equipped for high-risk babies, and counseling to prepare for a high-risk baby. To make such choices, more limited information on preferences will suffice, namely the functions that measure the relative losses in utility from receiving suboptimal treatment for each underlying condition. (See Keeney and Raiffa, 1976.) Therefore, rather than use utilities themselves in this analysis, our measure of performance was losses or disutilities compared with optimal treatment.

Failure to diagnose an NTD *in utero* results in the birth of a child with an unanticipated affliction. The loss from this failure is the difference in utility between a regular delivery of an infant with an NTD and the action that would have been taken with foreknowledge: for some women, an abortion; for others, the arrangement of specialized services for the newborn, of which the most critical are immediate medical and surgical interventions.

Our analysis considers two separate loss functions, one for women who would accept abortion, the other for women who would prepare. In each case—for convenience, but without loss of generality—we use a scale on which the disutility of correct diagnosis is 0 and the disutility of the worst error, not diagnosing spina bifida, is 1. Because an anencephalic newborn typically dies within a few days, foreknowledge makes less difference to either an "aborter" or a "preparer." Other errors are scaled in relation to those two extremes. Although the loss functions are quite different for the two groups, the numerical values assigned to outcomes have the same ordering and range. The losses of 1, for failure to diagnose spina bifida, are not comparable, however, since the ideal chosen outcomes would not have been the same for aborters and preparers.

In both scales (labeled "women who would abort" and "women who would prepare" in Table 6), the greatest disutility is associated with failure to diagnose spina bifida. To illustrate the process of scaling other errors (for example, aborting an unaffected fetus), consider a woman who would abort if the risk of a fetus with spina bifida were high enough. Let us say that she would just be willing to abort if that probability were p, offering a complementary probability 1 - p of a normal birth. Represent the loss of failing to abort a fetus with spina bifida as 1, and that of aborting an unaffected fetus as Y. Given that the expected losses balance, we must have $1 \times p = Y(1 - p)$, which implies that $Y = p/(1-p)$. If $p = 0.17$, for example, then $Y = 0.20$, the value used in our sample utility scale. On this scale, the loss from failing to abort a fetus with anencephaly is assigned a value of 0.10, only one-tenth the loss from failing to abort a fetus with spina bifida. This implies

Table 6
Losses from misdiagnosis in ELAs[a]

| | Type of Pregnancy | | | |
	Anencephaly	Spina Bifida	Unaffected	Multiple Gestation
Action	*Women Who Would Abort:*			
Abort (Terminate)	0.00	0.00	0.20	0.20
Continue Pregnancy	0.10	1.00	0.00	0.00
Action	*Women Who Would Prepare:*			
Prepare	0.00	0.00	0.10	0.10
Do Not Prepare	0.05	1.00	0.00	0.00

[a]Equivalent losses avoided.

that if anencephaly were the only risk of concern, a woman with these preferences would abort if the probability of anencephaly were above 2/3, the point at which the expected loss from abortion, $1/3 \times 0.20$, just balances the expected loss from risking anencephaly, $2/3 \times 0.10$.

For women who would accept abortion, misdiagnosing an unaffected or multiple-gestation fetus would lead to an unnecessary abortion in most cases. On the basis of a small informal poll—not of pregnant women—we assumed that this loss was 20 percent as serious as missing a case of spina bifida. This value is roughly consistent with the findings of a study of Down syndrome by Pauker, Pauker, and

Table 7
Outcomes of screening (number of women)[a]

| | Type of Pregnancy | | | | |
	Anencephaly	Spina Bifida	Unaffected	Multiple Gestation	Total
Total Number in Cohort	747	870	988,933	9,450	1,000,000
Alive at End of Testing	699	819	986,645	8,986	997,149
• No NTD Diagnosed	141	245	979,503	8,346	988,235
• Incomplete Testing	146	150	7,053	640	7,989
• NTD Diagnosed	412	424	89	0	925
Spontaneous Fetal Death	49	50	2,287	465	2,851
Cases Found by Screening	412	424	−89[b]	0	747

[a] "Alive at end of testing" and "spontaneous fetal death" sum to total number in cohort. The three rows with bullets sum to "alive at end of testing." "Cases found by screening" are the number of pregnancies diagnosed with NTDs. Elements may not sum exactly due to rounding.

[b] The negative number of unaffected pregnancies indicates that these pregnancies are misdiagnosed as affected by NTDs.

McNeil (1981). They asked 338 prospective parents in a health maintenance organization what minimum probability of an abnormality would prompt them to seek abortion. Although responses varied from probabilities of almost 0 to 100 percent, their median value was 20 percent and the mean was 33 percent.

For women who would respond to a positive NTD test result by preparing for the birth of an affected child, we calibrate their losses with a different question: what is the lowest probability that your fetus has a NTD at which you would prepare for the birth of an affected child? Preparation would include planning to deliver in a high-risk obstetrical facility, arranging for specialists to be available for testing and possible surgery, and receiving counseling on what to expect and how to cope with the stresses of a disabled or dying infant. We have no quantitative information on the distribution of benefits from early medical intervention for babies with spina bifida. Case studies reveal that the benefits can be substantial in some instances, including the avoidance of blindness, deafness or severe mental impairment.[8] Unnecessary preparation would create needless anxiety and inconvenience, which we count as a much smaller loss.

3. Results

Diagnostic success

Table 7 shows the diagnoses that would result from a screening program with the cutoff at the 95th percentile. At completion of screening, 925 women are diagnosed as having an NTD-affected fetus. That diagnosis is correct for 90 percent of these women. Excluding spontaneous fetal deaths, screening finds 59 percent of fetuses with anencephaly (412 out of 699); it identifies 52 percent of the fetuses with spina bifida (424 out of 819). These modest yields reflect principally the limited sensitivity of the first screening test, but also dropouts from testing. Unavoidably, some 89 unaffected fetuses in the cohort (about 1 in 11,000) are misdiagnosed as abnormal after complete screening.

Overall, our base case screening program correctly identifies 836 pregnancies with abnormalities—a bit over half of the cases of NTD actually present in the population—misdiagnoses 89 unaffected fetuses, and leaves 7,693 with incorrect positive findings based on incomplete testing. The societal value of these outcomes depends on the actions subsequently taken by the mothers, whose personal judgments of welfare are the ultimate benchmark. The sources of values for individuals depend on personal and ethical parameters, which are beyond the scope of this analysis.

It is more difficult to define the outcomes for the 7,989 women who fail to complete the testing program. Each receives a positive result on some interim screening test and declines to proceed with testing. For 296 women, the positive finding is correct: each of these fetuses is in fact affected by an NTD. For the remaining 7,693 women, the positive finding is incorrect: these fetuses are normal.[9]

Equivalent losses avoided (ELAs)

The total loss for the cohort is the actual disutility compared with a theoretical optimum of perfect knowledge (as if it were somehow known, at no cost, risk, or inconvenience, whether a fetus was affected by an NTD). Since individuals with different utilities could make different decisions, we alternatively applied each of the utility scales to the entire cohort. That is, we made two calculations, the first

81

Table 8

Cost-effectiveness results

Percentile Cutoff for First MSAFP	Equivalent Losses Avoided	Reduction (%)	Screening Cost ($)	Cost-Effectiveness ($/ELA)
Women Who Would Abort[a]				
99th[b]	351	39.4	$30,187,950	$86,006
95th	448	50.4	39,098,610	87,274
Increment	97	11.0	8,910,660	91,862
Women Who Would Prepare[c]				
99th[a]	334	39.0	29,310,750	87,757
95th	437	51.1	37,988,610	86,930
Increment	103	12.1	8,910,660	—[d]

[a] Potential Equivalent Losses Avoided (ELAs) are 890.

[b] Number of spontaneous fetal deaths (SFDs) in 99th percentile is rescaled to that in 95th percentile.

[c] Potential ELAs are 855.

[d] Incremental cost-effectiveness ratio is not applicable because the 95th percentile achieves more ELAs and costs less per ELA.

assuming that all women would choose to abort an affected fetus, the second assuming that all would choose to prepare for delivery of an affected child. As no process of aggregating or comparing losses across individuals with different types of preferences would be valid without the introduction of arbitrary assumptions, we made no attempts to combine the two groups.

We measured disutility on a scale where each unit represents the equivalent of the loss from failure to diagnose one case of spina bifida. The outcomes of the screening program for each group then are computed as equivalent losses avoided (ELA), using that group's scale. Note that the consequences of the error are quite different in the two cases: failing to abort for the aborters, failing to prepare for the preparers. Table 6 shows that the scalings for other errors are different for the two groups as well.

The success of the screening program in providing ELAs is shown in Table 8. The program in our basic analysis secures 50.4 percent of the maximum ELAs for the aborters and 51.1 percent of the maximum for the preparers.

Cost-effectiveness

Our basic cost-effectiveness analyses use the ratio of dollar costs to ELAs, which are the average costs of producing each equivalent loss avoided. To calculate these values, the total costs of screening and follow-up testing for the cohort are divided by the net gains to the cohort in equivalent losses avoided. At the 95th percentile cutoff, if all women chose to abort an affected fetus, the cost per ELA would be $87,274; for women who would prepare, the figure would be $86,930.

4. Discussion

Interpretations of cost-effectiveness findings

To interpret the cost-effectiveness values, they must be compared with a valuation of the importance society attaches to preventing or planning for (according to the mother's preferences) the birth of a baby with spina bifida. For a woman who would abort, one relevant benchmark is the discounted cost of medical, supportive, and rehabilitative care for a person affected by spina bifida. Propper (1986) briefly discusses costs of $40,000 to $50,000 per year, though surely those numbers must apply to relatively severe cases of spina bifida. Layde et al. (1979) estimate discounted lifetime medical costs of $17,452 in 1977 dollars. Their estimate is conservative, for they project median survival to be only two years, and they extrapolate treatment costs from a range of disabilities, many requiring less medical care than spina bifida. Updating these costs to 1983 dollars, which would require a multiple between 2 and 3, and allowing for the substantial gains in life expectancy of children with spina bifida, lifetime medical costs would almost certainly exceed the $87,274 cost per ELA.[10]

Cost savings in other supportive costs, including possible loss of earnings for the parents, would tilt the economic scale still further. In other words, it costs less to diagnose, and for aborters thus prevent, spina bifida than to care for a person with the condition. Thus, screening programs in which affected fetuses are aborted almost surely reduce net aggregate societal dollar costs for screening, treatment and care.

Some women would respond to the diagnosis of spina bifida by planning before delivery for intensive medical intervention at birth, as well as by getting counseling. Here again the findings of our analysis are useful in deciding whether a screening program should be undertaken, though they do not provide an unambiguous conclusion without the introduction of further value judgments. The question is whether starting intervention early, rather than several days after the birth of an infant, improves the prognosis of the infant and family enough to warrant an expenditure of up to $86,930 per infant so benefited.[11] Part of these medical costs might be offset by lifetime cost savings associated with early medical intervention. We could find no estimates of the dollar savings—or indeed possibly increased expenditures since life expectancy may be extended—due to early medical intervention.

The actual results of a screening program will depend on the relative sizes of the two subpopulations, aborters and preparers. To the extent that testing identifies affected fetuses whose mothers elect abortion, it will tend to save medical costs. Thus, on both measures we consider, a screening program is beneficial among women who would choose abortion; it saves societal dollars and leads to the mother's preferred outcome. If a woman would respond to a positive test result by preparing, rather than aborting the fetus, it is unlikely that savings in lifetime medical costs will outweigh costs of screening. If they do not, determining whether the program is worthwhile requires a comparison between health gain and the dollars required to produce it. In essence, we must determine whether the disability avoided throughout the lifetime of a child with spina bifida because of early medical intervention and counseling of the parents merits the expenditures entailed to diagnose an affected fetus.

Sensitivity analysis

What would be the effect of imposing a more stringent definition of abnormality in testing? We performed a sensitivity analysis assuming that the cutoff in the first MSAFP test was the 99th percentile score of unaffecteds, rather then the 95th percentile as in the base case.[12] Under this plan, fewer women would be identified as positive on the first screen, and so total program costs are moderately lower. (This change cannot reduce the costs of the first test, which are the highest in aggregate.)[13]

The cost-effectiveness ratio of the 95th percentile program for a potential aborter is less than 2 percent less favorable than that of the 99th percentile program (Table 8). The incremental cost-effectiveness ratio of going from the 99th percentile to the more inclusive 95th percentile, in turn, is only 5 percent more than that for 95th percentile screening. Under either program, for an aborter the cost per ELA is less than our estimate of the lifetime costs of care for a person with spina bifida.

Given that the 99th percentile program is slightly more cost-effective, it should be chosen if the amount of money available for this type of screening is so limited that we cannot offer it to all who would like to participate. However, if these programs are considered more than marginally worthwhile, and if on that basis dollars will be made available for them, then it seems virtually certain that the 95th percentile program should be chosen in preference. It offers 1.28 times as many ELAs for women who would abort.

For women who would prepare, the 95th percentile program has an even stronger claim for being preferred. It starts out by being more cost-effective than the 99th. It secures 1.29 times as many ELAs for these women. In summary, if society is launching a screening program in this area, it should use the 95th percentile cutoff on the first MSAFP in preference to the 99th, whether the program aims at aborters, preparers, or a population that is mixed. Its major advantage is that it enables society to purchase more of something worth buying, at a slightly higher per unit price for aborters and a slightly lower one for preparers.

Limitations and extensions of the analysis

Cost-effectiveness analysis has both strengths and limitations in its application to screening problems. It can clarify the elements of a complex clinical issue, describe the technical performance of a screening strategy, make underlying values explicit, and systematically test critical parameters. Our illustrative analysis also demonstrates the degree to which available data determine the policy implications of an analysis. Their accuracy and representativeness determine its validity.

In this instance, a major data limitation was the very limited information we had about individuals' preferences, for these preferences play a major role in our analysis. Fortunately, our major results are quite robust with respect to alternative preference structures. Once a woman has proceeded through all tests and has been told she is likely to have a fetus with an NTD, the likelihood that an NTD is present is extremely high. If ultrasonography has confirmed the original gestational age but has not found an NTD, and if amniotic fluid AFP is positive for NTDs (node 20A), the probability of an NTD is 77 percent (287/372). If ultrasonography and amniotic fluid AFP are both positive for NTDs (node 18A), that probability is 99 percent (549/554). To illustrate robustness for an aborter, suppose that the loss from an unnecessary abortion were as high as 3.33 times the loss of failing to abort a fetus with spina bifida (i.e., she would accept an abortion only if the likelihood of fetus with spina bifida were 75 percent), in contrast to the 0.20 times as high employed in this analysis. Abortion would still be her optimal action at the two nodes where the decision arises.

The loss functions for aborters and preparers in this analysis do not represent the expressed or revealed preferences of any actual group of pregnant women confronted with NTD testing; rather they are the opinion of a few individuals on how such women would be likely to feel. No group of women would present homogeneous values regarding prenatal testing, elective abortion, fetal treatment, and handicapped infants. If our assumed utilities in some sense represent an average for each group, our ELA computations and costs per ELA would be representative for each. If within each category individuals with heterogeneous utilities could make decisions that reflected their personal preferences, then the true gains to the programs would be even higher.

As we remarked earlier, further value judgments would be required to combine cost-effectiveness measures for aborters and preparers, since the maximum loss used for calibration—failing to take appropriate action for spina bifida—represents quite different outcomes in the two circumstances. Since the expected medical costs of the program are likely to be negative for aborters, it would seem that screening for this group is clearly justified. Though the justification is less immediate, it is conceivably even more justified for preparers. Such a determination would depend substantially on the assessment of and valuation of medical benefits to the child with spina bifida that return to preparation and early medical intervention. We have made no estimates of those values. In summary, a clear justification for prenatal NTD screening for women who would prepare cannot tumble out of our numbers, since we are presented with noncomparables, namely, screening expenditures versus limitations on disability. Assuming that the screening program provides medical benefits for preparers and has net dollar costs, it should be compared with other ways of purchasing health with dollars. The most relevant comparisons would be with other programs that provide benefits to newborns and their families. Provision of neonatal intensive care or nutrition programs for pregnant women are but two of many possible examples.

Classical cost-effectiveness analysis usually focuses on final outcomes; hence considerations of anxiety are excluded. The screening program we examined may influence a woman's well-being during pregnancy, increasing her concern that her fetus may be affected by an NTD or reassuring her that it is not. For some women, the very consideration of the testing process may raise to consciousness a problem of which they were previously unaware. As the results of each successive test become known, the woman's level of anxiety should rise or fall according to the change in her probability of having a baby with an NTD. Women with positive findings become more concerned, while those with negative results—the vast majority—are reassured.

If anxiety were a linear function of risk (that is, a given change in risk always corresponds to the same proportional change in anxiety), it could be easily incorporated in classical decision analysis. The losses should include both the event (such as NTD) and the fear of that event. However, levels of anxiety are not linear functions of risk; we therefore need a more complex psychological model of the way people experience changes in well-being. An alternative approach would view decision analysis as a useful normative technique to describe how people would and should react if they were completely informed, unemotional in their decisions, and "experienced" probabilities in proportion to their values (see Part II, Section B).

Some important considerations are omitted from this analysis, such as the ability to provide specialized services on a widespread basis; others, such as anxiety, are mentioned but not incorporated into our calculations. Perhaps the most important qualification is that many considerations are telescoped into the pregnant women's utility scale, such as the well-being of the fetus and newborn, and effects on all members of the family. Our analysis may underestimate the value of MSAFP screening because it does not consider that low MSAFP values are suggestive of increased risk of Down Syndrome; it also does not consider screening only groups at increased risk of NTDs. In the latter case, the actual yield from screening would be higher. Finally, we do not assess improvements in technology. As new tests become available, such as measuring AChE (fetal amniotic acetylcholinesterase) through amniocentesis, screening will become more accurate. New calculations, using the framework outlined in this paper, will be required to determine cost-effectiveness.

5. Conclusions

The major elements of a cost-effectiveness analysis include structuring of the decision problem (describing and ordering the choices and chance events), estimating or deriving the probabilities of each chance event, estimating monetary costs to the program under analysis, and assessing the utility (desirability) of each outcome. Because the monetary costs of screening are generally borne by society at large, while the emotional costs of aborting or giving birth fall heavily on the affected family, the two costs are considered separately.

Our base case screening program, using a cutoff at the 95th percentile for the first test, would identify 52 percent of the live fetuses with spina bifida (424 identified out of 819 present in a cohort of one million pregnant women) and 59 percent of the live fetuses with anencephaly (412 out of 699 in the cohort). It would mistakenly classify as abnormal 89 out of almost one million women with unaffected singleton or multiple-gestation pregnancies. It would also leave 7,989 women who discontinued testing with the thought that their fetuses might be affected with an NTD. Of these, 296 actually would be affected; 7,693 would be normal. The cost of this screening program was calculated to be $39 per participant, more than half of which is due to the initial MSAFP screening test. The state of California is charging $40 for its screening program (Propper, 1986).

Is this screening program worthwhile for the participants? To address this question, we first assumed that women who completed testing with a positive result would act as if their fetus were affected and seek abortion or prepare for a high-risk baby. Two utility scales were constructed, one for each group, to weigh the gains from identifying spina bifida and anencephaly against the losses from misdiagnosing unaffected fetuses.

In a program that emphasizes free choice, participants can always decide to ignore admittedly imperfect tests. Provided participants are fully informed and free to respond to information as they see best, any screening program must be beneficial or neutral on average *to them*. If the inconvenience, medical and financial costs to them were sufficient, not a likely problem with prenatal screening for NTDs, they might choose not to participate. Alternative loss functions could also be considered. For utility scales that assign a sufficiently heavy penalty to misclassifying a normal fetus, for example, prenatal screening for NTDs would be disadvantageous to a pregnant woman.

As we observed earlier, limitations on available data preclude a comprehensive numerical result. The results described here depend on both uncertain data and assumptions and because of their inherent limitations should be interpreted with care. We cannot provide answers to a number of important questions regarding the efficacy of NTD screening for the pregnant population, but our study was successful in applying cost-effectiveness analysis to a complex clinical issue. It yields important conclusions on some issues, and identifies the critical inputs required to reach conclusions on other issues.

To summarize our numerical results, for women who would prepare, the cost per ELA ranges from $87,000 to $90,000 depending on the first test cutoff. Such a program may be justified in terms of cost, depending on the valuation of the medical gains and the cost savings that may come from preparation and early medical intervention. Now that NTD screening programs are actually being used, research on the magnitude of these benefits becomes a priority issue.

For women who would abort and who accept the fact that testing will occasionally misdiagnose an unaffected pregnancy, this screening program not only increases their welfare, but saves economic resources. The cost per ELA ranges from $86,000 to $92,000 depending on the precise cutoff selected for continuing testing (Table 8). These costs seem likely to be outweighed by savings in lifetime costs of caretaking and medical treatment.

Our intent was to demonstrate that cost-effectiveness analysis provides a useful framework for organizing the information about preferences, probabilities, and costs needed to evaluate a screening program, and to describe the performance of the NTD test protocol. Our analysis developed an output measure, *dollar cost per ELA*, that assessed effectiveness as loss from optimal performance. This measure should serve a useful guidepost for policy in evaluating other medical interventions as well as NTD screening. For preparers, additional data—notably the implications of preparation for lifetime medical costs of a spina bifida child—and value judgments are required to determine whether the screening program is worthwile. For aborters, the screening program is worthwhile on both criteria employed: cost savings and the woman's self-assessed welfare.

Acknowledgements

The authors are grateful to Elena Nightingale, M.D., Ph.D., who directed the broader study of the role of analytic methods in prenatal diagnosis from which this work was derived and who carefully reviewed previous drafts of this manuscript. The authors are also grateful to Fredric Frigoletto, M.D., and to Frederick Mosteller, Ph.D., Nancy Jackson, and Jane Sisk, Ph.D., for valuable advice and comments.

6. Footnotes

[1]Cost estimates from Propper, 1986.

[2]Some women over 35 years of age might detect neural tube defects through an amniocentesis for Down syndrome. We assume no targeting of the program toward higher risk ethnic groups.

[3]If the ultrasonography is diagnostic of an NTD, the physician may recommend either an amniocentesis for confirmation or acceptance of the ultrasonographic diagnosis. In this analysis, we made the conservative assumption that all women with diagnostic ultrasonographic findings would be offered amniocentesis.

[4]If women worry about NTDs at all, on average, given the rarity of the condition, anxiety would be reduced, since more than 94 percent of women will have only negative tests.

[5]There are several reports on the relative risk of spontaneous miscarriage following amniocentesis. Some reports, such as Tabor et al. (1986), cite a higher relative risk (2.3) than the one used here.

[6]Jeremiah Mahoney, M.D., Yale Medical School, personal communication, June 1984.

[7]Abortion costs are the midpoint for clinics in the New York and Boston areas, adjusted to 1984 dollars. Planned Parenthood League of Massachusetts, personal communication, June 1986.

[8]See Nightingale and Meister, this volume, for a discussion of the benefits of preparation.

[9]For a woman who fails to complete testing, whether an aborter or preparer, the appropriate action given the preference structures specified in Table 6 is to continue with pregnancy, with one exception. Women who decline an amniocentesis after ultrasonography is positive, node 10B, have a 40 percent risk (135/337) of an NTD-affected fetus. They should abort or prepare. Our analysis assumes that they merely continue with pregnancy.

[10]The anencephaly cases would not offer substantial savings in medical costs. Since they make up roughly 10 percent of the expected losses avoided in our calculations, the actual breakeven number for medical costs would be roughly $95,000. That is, if children with spina bifida on average had lifetime medical costs of $95,000, this screening program would neither cost nor save dollars of medical expenditures. We do not consider the saved medical expenditures on unaffected fetuses mistakenly aborted, nor any earnings they would generate.

[11]Roughly 5 percent of these benefits are reaped for preparing for births of babies with anencephaly, where there are no gains from early medical intervention. Eliminating these from the analysis would give a figure of roughly $91,000 per correctly prepared-for baby with spina bifida. Preparing for a mistakenly diagnosed child who turns out to be unaffected incurs no substantial medical costs in the aggregate.

[12]If the same test is to be repeated, and a woman is classified as positive if her result is above the cutoff both times, the power of the test will be greatest if both cutoffs are set at the same level. (As a secondary consideration, setting the first cutoff slightly more stringently and the second one less stringently will save some costs of second tests.)

[13]To compare results from the 99th and 95th percentile tests, it was necessary to rescale downward the number of equivalent losses by the factor 890/904. This correction is necessary because spontaneous fetal deaths are counted only through completion of the screening program. The 99th percentile program eliminates women sooner from screening, so only 1,007 spontaneous fetal deaths are counted, compared with 2,852 under the 95th percentile test.

7. References

Department of Health and Human Services. *Diagnostic ultrasound imaging in pregnancy: Report of a consensus conference*. Washington: Superintendent of Documents. 1984 (NIH Publication No. 84-667).

Gardner S., Burton B.K. and Johnson A.M. Maternal serum alpha-fetoprotein screening: A report of the Forsyth County Project. *American Journal of Obstetrics and Gynecology* 1981, *140*, 250-253.

Goldberg, M.F. and Oakley G.P. Prenatal screening for anencephaly-spina bifida: Some epidemiological projections for a national program. In Porter, I.H. and Hook, E.B. (Eds.) *Service and education in medical genetics*. New York: Academic Press, 1979.

Grace, H.J. Prenatal screening for neural tube defects in South Africa. An assessment. *South African Medical Journal*, 1981, *60*, 324-329.

Hagard, S., Carter, F., and Milner, R. Screening for spina bifida cystica. *British Journal of Preventive and Social Medicine*, 1976, *30*, 40-53.

Hibbard, B.M., Roberts, C.J., Elder, G.H., Evans, K.T., and Laurence, K.M. Can we afford screening for neural tube defects? The South Wales experience. *British Medical Journal*, 1985, *290*, 295-297.

Keeney, R.L. and Raiffa, H. *Decisions with multiple objectives: Preferences and value trade-offs*. New York: John Wiley and Sons, 1976.

Layde, P.M., von Allmen, S.D., and Oakley, G.P. Maternal serum alpha-fetoprotein screening: A cost-benefit analysis. *American Journal of Public Health*, 1979, *69*, 566-573.

Macri, J.N., Haddow, J.E., and Weiss, R.R. Screening for neural tube defects in the United States: A summary of the Scarborough conference. *American Journal of Obstetrics and Gynecology* 1979a, *133*, 119-125.

Macri, J.N., Weiss, R.R., and Libster, B. Maternal serum alpha-fetoprotein screening for neural tube defects: Structure and organization. In Porter, I.H. and Hook, E.B. (Eds.) *Service and education in medical genetics*. New York: Academic Press, 1979b.

National Center for Health Statistics: Advance report of final natality statistics, 1980. *Monthly Vital Statistics Report*: November 30, 1982, 1-8.

National Institute of Child Health and Human Development (NICHHD) National Registry for Amniocentesis Study Group: Midtrimester amniocentesis for prenatal diagnosis: safety and accuracy. *Journal of the American Medical Association*, 1976, *236*, 1471-1476.

Nelson, L.H. Neural tube defects. Paper presented at the 1983 AIUM/SDMS Annual Convention, New York, October 1983.

Pauker, S.G., Pauker, S.P. and McNeil, B.J. The effect on private attitudes of public policy. *Medical Decision Making* 1981, *1*, 103-114.

Propper, L. Alpha-fetoprotein screening program begun. *American Medical News*. 1986, p. 13.

Roberts, C.J., et al. Diagnostic effectiveness of ultrasound in detection of neural tube defects. *Lancet*, 1983, *1*, 1068-1069

Sadovnick, A.D. and Baird, P.A. A cost-benefit analysis of a population screening programme for neural tube defects. *Prenatal Diagnosis*, 1983, *3*, 117-126.

Shepard, D.S., Meister, S.J., and Zeckhauser, R.J. Screening for neural tube defects: An application of decision analysis. In *Health interventions and population heterogeneity: Evidence from Japan and the U.S.* NIRA output, NRF-83-1. Tokyo, Japan: National Institute for Research Advancement, 1985, pp. 69-89.

Tabor, A., Madsen, M., Obel, E.B., et al. Randomized controlled trial of genetic amniocentesis in 4604 low-risk women. *Lancet*, 1986, *1*, 1287-1292.

8. Appendixes

Table A1
Performance of screening protocol:
Explanations and sources of data

Group	Explanation
0	According to the results of the MSAFP, Group 0 is sorted into Group 1 (elevated MSAFP), 2 (normal MSAFP), or 3 (low MSAFP).
1	We followed Goldberg and Oakley (1979) and used the 95th percentile as the cutoff for abnormal MSAFP. Thus, the sensitivity for anencephaly is .88, the sensitivity for spina bifida is .78 and the specificity is .95—and we assumed all multiple gestations would have false positives. Therefore, Group 1 includes 88% of the fetuses with anencephaly, 78% of those with spina bifida, 5% of the unaffected fetuses, and all of the multiple gestations.
1A	The women in Group 1 are offered a repeat MSAFP. Group 1A accepts the repeat MSAFP and continues in the screening program. Our rates for accepting and declining are the average of the rates reported by Macri et al. (1979a,1979b).
1B	Group 1B declines and these women make decisions about their pregnancies.
2	Group 2 includes 12% of the fetuses with anencephaly, 22% of the fetuses with spina bifida, and 93% of the unaffected fetuses. Group 2 is considered free of NTD; these women have completed screening and decided about their pregnancies (continue to term, prepare or terminate).
3	Group 3, following Nelson (1983), also stops screening. We used Nelson's (1983) report on low MSAFP values to determine that Group 3 would include 1.7% of the unaffected fetuses. We assumed that this small group is unaffected by NTD, although errors in gestational age, fetal death and other disorders may be present.
4	Group 1A becomes Group 4.
5	Following Goldberg and Oakley (1979), the repeat MSAFP test has a sensitivity of .99 for anencephaly and spina bifida, and will correct 33.3 % of false positives among unaffected singletons. We assumed that 99% of multiple gestations would repeat their previous false positives. Therefore, Group 5 (elevated MSAFP) includes 99% of the fetuses with anencephaly and spina bifida that had elevations in the first MSAFP. It also includes 66.7% of the unaffected fetuses and 99% of the multiple gestations with a false positive on the initial MSAFP. Group 5 is offered ultrasonography.
5A	We averaged the rates of declining reported by Macri et al. (1979a, 1979b).
5B	and Gardner (1981) to estimate the sizes of Group 5A (accept ultrasonography) and Group 5B (decline ultrasonography). The same authors reported rates of spontaneous fetal death at this point in testing; again, we averaged the rates.
5C	Group 5C is the group that has had a second elevated MSAFP, accepted the next test and not experienced spontaneous fetal death. These women receive ultrasonography.
5D	Group 5D is like Group 5C, except they experience spontaneous fetal death.
5E	Group 5E has had a second elevated MSAFP, declined the next test and not experienced spontaneous fetal death.
5F	Group 5F is like Group 5E, except they experience spontaneous fetal death. The women in Group 5E stop screening and make decisions about their pregnancies.
6	Group 6 (normal repeat MSAFP) includes 1% of the fetuses with anencephaly and spina bifida, 33.3% of the unaffected fetuses and 1% of the multiple gestations. Women in Group 6 complete testing and make decisions about their pregnancies.
7	Group 7 (Group 5C from Figure 3) is first split into viable fetus (Group 8) and fetal

Performance of screening protocol:
Explanations and sources of data

8	death (Group 9). The rate of fetal death (3.31%) is the average of those reported by
9	Macri et al. (1979a, 1979b) and Gardner (1981). Group 8 is then split, according to whether or not the ultrasonography produces a visible NTD, Group 10 is apparent NTD.
10	Group 10 is the group with NTDs apparent during ultrasonography. We used Goldberg and Oakley's (1979 et al.) estimate that 99% of anencephaly would be visualized, and Roberts et al. (1983) report that 33.3% of spina bifida would be visualized. Roberts also reported that 3.94% of unaffected fetuses would be mistakenly thought to have NTDs. We assumed that no multiple gestations would be classified into Group 10. This leaves 1% of fetuses with anencephaly, 66.7% of fetuses with spina bifida, and 96.06% of unaffected fetuses in Group 11. It also carries the multiple gestations in Group 8 into Group 11.
10A 10B	We assumed that even after an NTD was visualized on ultrasonography examination, the woman would be offered amniocentesis to confirm the finding. As with all tests, some women decline (Group 10B) and stop testing. The remainder (Group 10A) go on to have amniocentesis. The rate of declining was taken from Nelson (1983).
11	Group 11 is fetuses with no NTD apparent at ultrasonography.
12 13	The group (Group 11) where no NTD has been visualized is split according to presence of multiple gestation (Group 12) or singleton pregnancy (Group 13). Following the NIH Consensus Panel (1984), we assumed that all multiple gestations would be found and that no singleton pregnancies would be mistakenly considered to be multiple. Group 13, then, is a group where the fetus is a viable singleton and no NTD has been visualized.
14	The final contribution of ultrasonography is to verify or correct the estimate of gestational age. If the age is corrected (Group 14), we assumed that the previous MSAFP values would be reclassified as normal rather than elevated. These women complete testing and make decisions about their pregnancies. The rate defining this group (23.6% of unaffected fetuses) is the average of rates reported by Macri et al. (1979a, 1979b) and Gardner (1981).
15	The remainder of Group 13 becomes Group 15—the group that has gestational age verified, confirming that previous MSAFP values were elevated. Group 15 is offered amniocentesis.
15A 15B	Some women decline amniocentesis (Group 15B) and stop testing. The remainder (Group 15A) accept and go on to have amniocentesis. The rate of declining (17.617%) is taken from Nelson (1983).
16 17	Groups 16 and 17 have amniocentesis and are split according to AFP results, i.e., normal or elevated.
18 19 20 21	We used Goldberg and Oakley's findings about sensitivity and specificity to define these groups. The elevated AFP groups (Groups 18 and 20) include 90% of the fetuses with anencephaly and spina bifida, and 0.5% of unaffected fetuses. The normal AFP groups (Groups 19 and 21) include 10% of fetuses with anencephaly and spina bifida and 99.5% of unaffected fetuses.
18A 19A 20A 21A	Groups 18A, 19A, 20A, 21A have viable fetuses and have completed all screening tests; two of them (Group 18A and 20A) have finished screening with a complete series of positive findings. The other two (Group 19A and 21A) have finished screening with a negative finding. All four groups of women now make decisions about their pregnancies.
18B 19B 20B 21B	Groups 18, 19, 20 and 21 are then diminished by spontaneous fetal death. Following the NICHHD (1976) findings, we assumed a 3.5% fetal death rate, defining Groups 18B, 19B, 20B, 21B.

Table A2

Formulas used in calculations (Base Case)[a]

	Type of Fetus			
	Anencephaly	Spina Bifida	Unaffected	Multiple Gestation
Group				
0	747	870	988933	9450
1	0.88*(G0)	0.78*(G0)	0.05*(G0)	G0
1A	0.9483*(G1)	0.9483*(G1)	0.9483*(G1)	0.9483*(G0)
1B	0.0517*(G1)	0.0517*(G1)	0.0517*(G1)	0.0517*(G1)
2	0.12*(G0)	0.22*(G0)	0.9334*(G0)	0
3	0	0	0 .166*(G0)	0
4	(G1A)	(G1A)	(G1A)	(G1A)
5	0.99*(G4)	0.99*(G4)	0.667*(G4)	0.99*(G4)
5A	0.98263*(G5)	0.98263*(G5)	0.98263*(G5)	0.98263*(G5)
5B	0.01737*(G5)	0.01737*(G5)	0.01737*(G5)	0.01737*(G5)
5C	0.97947*(G5A)	0.97947*(G5A)	0.97947*(G5A)	0.97947*(G5A)
5D	0.02053*(G5A)	0.02053*(G5A)	0.02053*(G5A)	0.02053*(G5A)
5E	0.97947*(G5B)	0.97947*(G5B)	0.97947*(G5B)	0.97947*(G5B)
5F	0.02053*(G5B)	0.02053*(G5B)	0.02053*(G5B)	0.02053*(G5B)
6	0.01*(G4)	0.01*(G4)	0.333*(G4)	0.01*(G4)
7	(G5C)	(G5C)	(G5C)	(G5C)
8	0.9669*(G7)	0.9669*(G7)	0.9669*(G7)	0.9669*(G7)
9	0.0331*(G7)	0.0331*(G7)	0.0331*(G7)	0.0331*(G7)
10	0.99*(G8)	0.333*(G8)	0.0394*(G8)	0
10A	0.82383*(G10)	0.82383*(G10)	0.82383*(G10)	0.82383*(G10)
10B	0.17617*(G10)	0.17617*(G10)	0.17617*(G10)	0.17617*(G10)
11	0.01*(G8)	0.667*(G8)	0.9606*(G8)	(G8)
12	0	0	0	(G11)
13	(G11)	(G11)	(G11)	0
14	0	0	0.23603*(G13)	0
15	(G13)	(G13)	0.76397*(G13)	0
15A	0.82383*(G15)	0.82383*(G15)	0.82383*(G15)	0
15B	0.17617*(G15)	0.17617*(G15)	0.17617*(G15)	0
16	(G10A)	(G10A)	(G10A)	0
17	(G15A)	(G15A)	(G15A)	0
18	0.9*(G16)	0.9*(G16)	0.005*(G16)	0
18A	0.965*(G18)	0.965*(G18)	0.965*(G18)	0
18B	0.035*(G18)	0.035*(G18)	0.035*(G18)	0
19	0.1*(G16)	0.1*(G16)	0.995*(G16)	0
19A	0.965*(G19)	0.965*(G19)	0.965*(G19)	0
19B	0.035*(G19)	0.035*(G19)	0.035*(G19)	0
20	0.9*(G17)	0.9*(G17)	0.005*(G17)	0
20A	0.965*(G20)	0.965*(G20)	0.965*(G20)	0
20B	0.035*(G20)	0.035*(G20)	0.035*(G20)	0
21	0.1*(G17)	0.1*(G17)	0.995*(G17)	0
21A	0.965*(G21)	0.965*(G21)	0.965*(G21)	0
21B	0.035*(G21)	0.035*(G21)	0.035*(G21)	0

[a] Each group shown in Figures 2-5 is listed as a row in this Table. Each column shows the formula for one of the four types of fetuses. The expressions listed in parentheses are references to Groups, and each formula is column-specific. For example, the formula for Group 1, fetuses with anencephaly, reads 0.88*(G0) and means that Group 1, Anencephalic fetuses is 88% of Group 0. Thus, each term in parentheses refers to a group number of the type of fetus listed in that column. The sources for the formulas are given in Table A1.

Table A3
Number of women in each group [a]

Group	Anencephaly	Spina Bifida	Unaffected	Multiple Gestation	Sum (Row)
Group 0	747	879	988933	9450	100000
Group 1	657	679	49447	9450	60233
Group 1A	623	644	46890	8961	57119
Group 1B	34	35	2556	489	3114
Group 2	90	191	923070	0	923351
Group 3	0	0	16416	0	16416
Group 4	623	644	46890	8961	57119
Group 5	617	637	31276	8872	41402
Group 5A	606	626	30733	8718	40683
Group 5B	11	11	543	154	719
Group 5C	594	613	30102	8539	39847
Group 5D	12	13	631	179	835
Group 5E	10	11	532	151	704
Group 5F	0	0	11	3	15
Group 6	6	6	15614	90	15717
Group 7	594	613	30102	8539	39847
Group 8	574	593	29105	283	38529
Group 9	20	20	996	0	1319
Group 10	569	197	1147	0	1913
Group 10A	468	163	945	0	1576
Group 10B	100	35	202	8526	337
Group 11	6	395	27958	8256	36616
Group 12	0	0	0	0	8256
Group 13	6	395	27958	0	28360
Group 14	0	0	6599	0	6599
Group 15	6	395	21359	0	21761
Group 15A	5	326	17597	0	17927
Group 15B	1	70	3763	0	3834
Group 16	468	163	945	0	1576
Group 17	5	326	17597	0	17927
Group 18	422	146	5	0	573
Group 18A	407	141	5	0	553
Group 18B	15	5	0	0	20
Group 19	47	16	940	0	1003
Group 19A	45	16	907	0	968
Group 19B	2	1	33	0	35
Group 20	4	293	88	0	385
Group 20A	4	283	85	0	372
Group 20B	0	10	3	0	13
Group 21	0	33	17509	0	17542
Group 21A	0	32	16896	0	16928
Group 21B	0	1	613	0	614

[a] The size of each Group was calculated using our base case formulas in Table A2.